BODY, LAND AND SPIRIT

Janice Reid is a science graduate in geology from the University of Adelaide. She worked as a high-school teacher in Papua New Guinea before taking up a fellowship at the University of Hawaii in 1969 to study anthropology. In 1971 she began work on her doctorate in medical anthropology at Stanford University. Her speciality is the anthropology of health, medical care, and therapeutic systems of non-Western societies. In 1978, Dr Reid travelled extensively throughout Australia as a specialist adviser to the House of Representatives Standing Committee on Aboriginal Affairs during its inquiry into Aboriginal health. Since 1979 she has held the positions of Associate Professor in Medical Anthropology at the Department of Public Health, Sydney University and head of the School of Community Health at the Cumberland College of Health Sciences.

BODY, LAND AND SPIRIT

HEALTH AND HEALING IN ABORIGINAL SOCIETY

Edited by Janice Reid

University of Queensland Press

First published 1982 by University of Queensland Press,
Box 42, St Lucia, Queensland 4067 Australia
Reprinted in paperback 1984, 1989

Printed in Australia by The Book Printer, Melbourne

Distributed in the USA and Canada by
International Specialized Book Services, Inc.,
5602 N.E. Hassalo Street, Portland, Oregon 97213-3640

Cataloguing in Publication Data

National Library of Australia

Body, land and spirit

First published: St. Lucia, Qld.: University of Queensland Press, 1982.
Includes bibliographies.

[1]. Aborigines, Australian — Health and hygiene — Addresses, essays, lectures. [2]. Aborigines, Australian — Medical care — Addresses, essays, lectures. [3]. Aborigines, Australian — Medicine — Addresses, essays, lectures. 4. Medical anthropology — Australia — Addresses, essays, lectures. 5. Medicine, Primitive — Australia — Addresses, essays, lectures. I. Reid, Janice, 1947- .

362.1

ISBN 0 7022 1779 4

Contents

List of Contributors

Diane Bell, Department of Prehistory and Anthropology, Australian National University, Canberra, A.C.T.

Catherine H. Berndt, Department of Anthropology, University of Western Australia, Nedlands, W.A.

David Biernoff, Department of Behavioural Sciences, Darling Downs Institute of Advanced Education, Toowoomba, Qld.

Maggie Brady, Department of Psychiatry, Medical School, Flinders University of South Australia, Bedford Park, S.A.

Gillian Cowlishaw, Department of Social Sciences, Mitchell College of Advanced Education, Bathurst, N.S.W.

Annette Hamilton, Behavioural Sciences, Macquarie University, North Ryde, N.S.W.

Betty Meehan, Department of Prehistory, Research School of Pacific Studies, Australian National University, Canberra, A.C.T.

Rodney Morice, Mental Health Services Commission of Tasmania, Hobart, Tas.

Janice Reid, Commonwealth Institute of Health, Sydney University, N.S.W.

Neville Scarlett, Department of Botany, LaTrobe University, Bundoora, Vic.

Myrna Tonkinson, Australian Institute of Aboriginal Studies, Canberra, A.C.T.

Jack Waterford, *Canberra Times*, Canberra City, A.C.T.

Neville White, Department of Genetics and Human Variation, LaTrobe University, Bundoora, Vic.

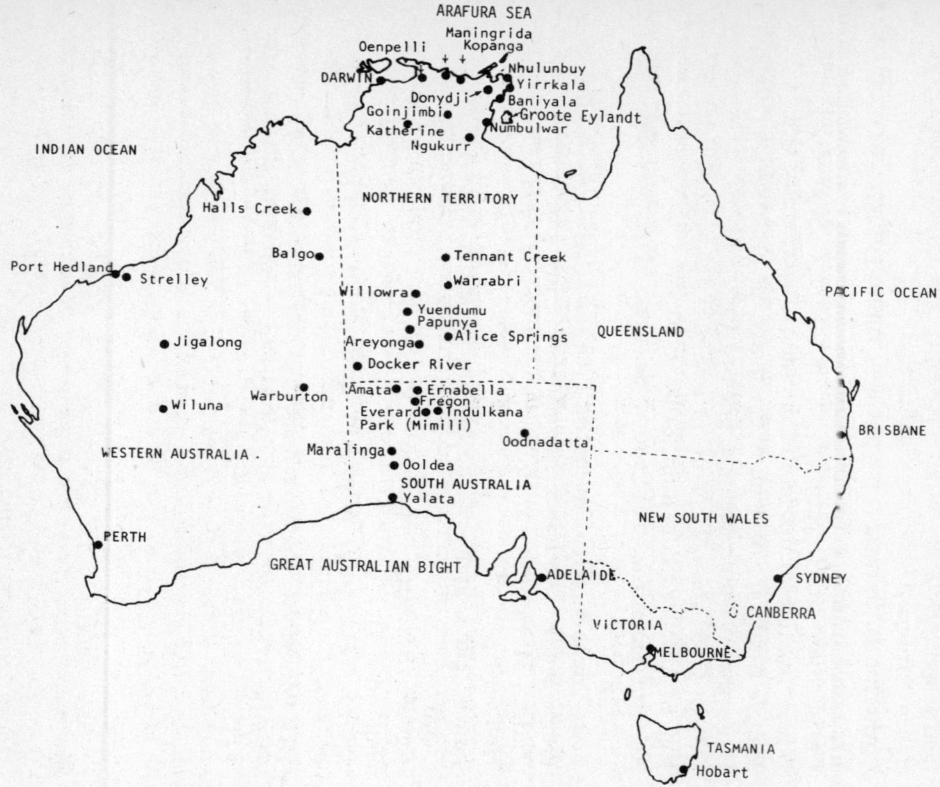

Map 1. Australia: Aboriginal Communities Referred to in Text.

Introduction
"The Australian Problem"

Janice Reid

In the year 2070, the first chroniclers were beginning to record the dimensions of "the Australian problem". Their accounts began in 2020, when the forces from the north landed in strength on Australia's shores, and the country capitulated. The foreigners closed Australia's parliaments, social services, business houses, schools, churches, theatres and sports-fields, transferred all private property to their own immigrant settlers, and permanently relocated the entire Australian population in tent encampments in the arid country areas.

By the time the Australians attracted the interest and concern of the chroniclers, their camps were in dispirited disarray. Ragged and rotting tents scarred the landscape. Although fifty years had passed since their establishment, the camps had none of the water, sewerage, sanitation or garbage-disposal facilities of the towns. The rations, available from distribution points in exchange for work tokens, were polished rice and weekly supplements of vegetables. Inspectors from the Health Ministry were concerned at the prevalence of malnutrition, gastroenteritis, anaemia, leprosy, tuberculosis, parasite infestations and respiratory tract infections. The lifestyle conditions such as diabetes and cardiovascular disease contributed heavily to the premature mortality of the adult population. The babies generally were dying from acute infections.

Emotional illness was widespread. Even the relatively well-balanced Australians — among them former doctors, teachers, managers, tradespeople, politicians and students — passed the days in a depressed malaise, or buoyed up by intoxicants or the transient excitement of games of chance. There was some discussion among the authorities about whether the high suicide rate and psychological disorders were products of the Australian culture or were a post-invasion phenomenon. Most experts favoured a cultural explanation and rejected suggestions that the stresses of camp life might be implicated.

Early on, some camp-dwellers had aspired to lead and organize community improvement campaigns, but lost interest when officials, while giving their blessing, refused to relinquish control of any administrative or political functions. Field officers of the Department of Australian

Advancement made many attempts to solicit the co-operation of the Australians in running projects devised by the Ministry for the betterment of the camps. The populace, however, evinced little interest in dog-farming, medicinal-herb cultivation and dry-rice agriculture. The Australians continued to reminisce perversely among themselves about study, books, free enterprise, salaries and job promotion.

The officials were kindly, but bewildered. They regretted the violent excesses of the early days of the invasion, but they could not understand the present recalcitrance of the Australians; their indifference to the government's exhortations to work the fields and improve themselves. Only the children, many of whom had no patience for the memories, values or traditions of their elders, had mastered the new tonal language and its alphabet of characters. Their English-speaking parents seemed either unable or unwilling to master these simple skills themselves. The adults consistently resisted the adoption of the introduced language, culture or agrarian lifestyle. They also undermined official efforts to recruit the young to a new ideology by covertly teaching them Australian history, English literature, writing and arithmetic. Even more troubling was the failure of the people to embrace the state religion, a synthesis of Hindu and Buddhist theologies. Most Australians irrationally retained more primitive Christian or agnostic beliefs and seemed foolishly unconcerned about their own enlightenment.

The spirit of the camps was no less a concern to administrative staff. They deplored the internecine strife among camp segments, and extolled the virtues of co-operation between families, whether or not they had known each other or come from the same social strata before settlement. And they despaired of the propensity of residents to "go wandering" from camp to camp for no apparent reason, or, at best, to join relatives for archaic festivals, which the Australians called "birthdays" and "Christmas". Perhaps the most disruptive force within the camps was the core of people who talked about their former houses, suburbs and jobs, and about "going home". These "fomenters" were few in number, and so were watchfully left alone. However, the young dissident settlers in the towns who agitated for "home rights" for the Australians were subject to the attentions of security services.

One of the government's greatest concerns was health. The new leaders were discomforted by discussions in the World Assembly about the inferior health status of subject peoples and the frequent references to Australians. They argued strenuously that every effort had been made to promote health, that the infant mortality rate was now only four times the national average, and that the average life expectancy was only ten to twenty years shorter. Everything that a health service could do had been done — even to training some medical assistants to give out medicines, weigh babies and dress sores. The residual morbidity and mortality, they insisted, was the result of the conditions in the camps, which were not their responsibility, and the deleterious customs of the Australians.

The initiatives of health authorities, the government explained to its overseas critics, were being undermined on several fronts. Illicit bands of doctors and nurses (pre-invasion professions no longer recognized) moved among the tents at night, tending the sick. The patients often failed to come to camp aid stations, where excellent practitioners from the mother country offered medical care. Most people seemed unable to grasp the principles of disease causation, patiently explained (though not in English) by the health educators. They did not, or could not, appreciate the logic of the elemental theory of disease (the bodily balance of earth, fire, air and water) and clung doggedly to a belief in "germs", "public health", "physiological dysfunction" and such mystical entities as "cancer". Indeed, in all ways, the Australians, through ignorance or defiance, thwarted efforts to help them.

It was generally agreed that governments can only help those who will help themselves: until the Australians recognized the manifest benefits of the post-2020 civilization and its medicine, the "Australian problem" would continue to challenge the nation . . .[1]

It has been said that Western medicine's epitaph will be that it was "brilliant in its scientific discoveries, superb in its technological breakthroughs, but woefully inept in its application of knowledge to those most in need".[2] This book is about one of the world's societies most in need: the Australian Aborigines. It explores the social and ecological disjunctions that have eroded their health, the traditional knowledge and resources that supported health and guided healing, and the ways Aborigines are dealing with the changes imposed on them.

Since Europeans colonized Australia, Aboriginal health has been the subject of government inquiries, political rhetoric, learned dissertations and classroom exercises. Assaults on the "Aboriginal health problem" have been directed by health departments, specialist teams, missions and Aboriginal health services. But in Australia of the late twentieth century, as in the apocryphal Australia of the late twenty-first, Aborigines remain the sickest people in Australia — a developing nation within a developed country.

Why? What are the authorities doing wrong? Is it fair to say, as an eminent physician said of one state health department, "If Aborigines were animals, the R.S.P.C.A. would prosecute"? Is health the responsibility of health authorities? If not, who is at fault? The white Australian settlers and their descendants? The Aborigines? Is it, perhaps, true that the Aborigines' diet, their culture and their lifestyle are inimical to good health?

The answers to these questions are as complex as the alarming patterns of morbidity and mortality they seek to explain. The closer one looks at the high rates of sickness and death in Aboriginal communities, the harder it becomes to discern causes, to design interventions or to attribute gains. What one looks for determines what one sees. Doctors, nurses or health planners tend to focus on medical services, nutrition, housing, public utilities or preventive health measures. Anthropologists note the attrition of the authority structures, religious life and social controls, which gave form and integrity to traditional Aboriginal society, the alienation of land, and the stresses of life on crowded missions and settlements. Historians explain the health troubles of the present in terms of the insults of the past: the early introduction of diseases such as smallpox and measles, which decimated some populations, the massacres (which continued well into the 1920s), the relocation of healthy, independent people on to ill-serviced settlements, and the confused and conflicting interests that have shaped policy towards Aborigines. All are, within the limitations of their perspectives, right. The current patterns of Aboriginal morbidity and mortality are the product of a constellation of historical, social, structural, economic and political forces.[3] The breadth and diversity of these forces makes it impossible to attribute blame or locate responsibility in a simple way.

At one level, the criticisms made of health authorities are justified. Historically, they were responsible for transposing a medical system developed in the cities of the Western, industrial world to a people who shared neither the culture, the disease profile nor the aspirations of white Australians. Health professionals failed to see that their medical practices and institutions were shaped not only by Western theories of illness and modes of treatment but also by Western values and social forms. The European cultural trappings of medical practice had no meaning to Aborigines. Conversely, Aboriginal perceptions of health and illness and indigenous curing systems were not recognized by health personnel, and so had little influence on their behaviour or programmes. The failure of health services to adapt to Aboriginal beliefs and mores created a "cultural chasm"[4] between services and users that, at best, thwarted mutual understanding and, at worst, made seeking treatment a frightening or mortifying experience for Aborigines.[5]

Not only culturally, but professionally, health services for Aborigines often marched to the beat of their own drummers. Health departments were unable to resist the political pressures for visible facilities and the professional interests that promoted them, and built hospitals and health centres, recruited more and better doctors and nurses, and stepped up detection and treatment programmes. Realizing in the 1970s that these were not very effective, several services trained Aboriginal health workers, expanded community programmes, experimented with health education and adopted a more permissive approach to traditional Aboriginal healers. Some functions of the services changed, but the structures that hindered radical change and innovation did not.

In general, the government institutions set up to deal with Aboriginal needs and problems are a pale blessing. The very structures that are designed to give health care, build houses, encourage enterprise, provide welfare, educate children and create jobs tend to foster dependency and undermine initiative. Aborigines become trapped by these structures in the role of client (or, occasionally, employee), unable to influence the processes or priorities of the institutions, whether or not they coincide with their own aspirations. At the same time, the professional interests of the staff act as a brake on "Aboriginalization". The health professions may be willing to see a cadre of Aboriginal health workers trained for supervised, grass-roots work. They often resist the idea, though, that such auxiliaries should have their own career paths and graduate to policy and executive positions.[6] In health, as elsewhere, Aborigines are subject to the culturally uninformed decisions of health staff, who come and go with confusing rapidity and are reluctant to relinquish responsibility. The Aboriginal health worker often feels trapped and becomes discouraged. Community determination is espoused as a goal, but is not experienced by Aborigines as a reality.

Further, government structures, usually bureaucratic departments, have their own cultures and demand certain forms of behaviour from the people they employ. As scholars from the time of Weber have explained, even if the people in bureaucracies care deeply about the plight of their clients, they must adhere to procedures that may have little to do with the problems to hand. Promotion and tenure depend on conformity to the policies of the institution, not on satisfaction of the needs of clients. Staff must account primarily to their superiors and to politicians for their expenditure and programmes. Thus financial resources are deployed in a way that satisfies accountants and administrators but may not satisfy or help Aborigines. In fact, in the health sector, the "spending on Aboriginal health" is largely spending on European staff salaries and on capital works, which may or may not have an impact on Aboriginal health and which certainly do not channel money into the local economy of Aboriginal communities, where it is most needed.

The issue is broader still than the inhibiting institutional framework of health care. The crucial question is: Do health services deliver health? Most doctors and nurses who have worked in Aboriginal communities, not to mention the Aborigines themselves, know they do not. Physical and emotional well-being also depend on the adequate provision of water, power, sewerage, housing and education, and on less tangible but equally important factors such as secure land tenure, social cohesion, cultural integrity and financial support. But to be "adequate", services to Aboriginal communities must do more than simply meet the technological and cost criteria applied in Australian towns and cities. They must be based on the priorities and views of Aborigines about their own health needs and give Aborigines the responsibility for their own development.

A philosophy of Aboriginal control obviously would constitute a radical change in Aboriginal health care. European agencies seem chronically unable to give the opinions, culture and organizing skills of Aborigines the central place in their programmes. Most health planning has been based on the medical model of service provision. This model is hierarchical, technology-dependent, centralized, professional and curative. Programmes are designed for people, rather than by them. This approach has so dominated thinking in Australia that authorities generally have ignored alternative approaches to health care that have developed elsewhere in the world during the last two decades as a reaction to the shortcomings of the medical model. These new approaches to health care vary from country to country[7] and take different forms[8] but embrace the same principles. These principles are generally subsumed by the label "primary health care".

Primary health care was endorsed by the member countries of the World Health Organization at its international conference in 1978, as the basis for achieving the aim of "health for all by the year 2000".[9] This approach is not simply a modification of the medical model; it is entirely different. Primary health care is integrated with other sectors, emphasizes prevention in its broadest sense, promotes health through environmental improvement and economic development, utilizes traditional healing resources, is based in the community, and is substantially planned and run by the "clients" themselves.

In Australia, the spirit of primary health care is most nearly captured not by government departments but by the Aboriginal Medical Services. These services are relatively autonomous, separately funded and community-based. Their directors and staff, a large proportion of whom are Aboriginal, see their role not only as providers of medical care but as health promoters and facilitators of community development projects outside the customary province of a medical service. It is no coincidence that some of the people actively involved in Aboriginal Medical Services also are assisting in legal and social reforms and land rights campaigns. The ends these services espouse — community health and autonomy — can be realized through the primary health care approach only if the philosophy is applied in its broadest sense.

As the founders of the Aboriginal Medical Services realized, the bones of any successful health innovation have to be fleshed out with people and plans that are meaningful to the participants and unequivocally acknowledge their stated needs. Further innovations in health care for Aborigines will have to be based on a clear perception of the causes of Aboriginal ill-health, of the unique resources that Aborigines themselves can bring to the endeavour, and of the introduced and indigenous strategies they already employ to deal with illness.

This book has been compiled to provide a framework within which health personnel, social planners and others can consider the crucial relationships between Aboriginal health, culture, social change and the structures of health care. It focuses on traditionally oriented communities[10] and draws together the experiences and observations of individuals who have lived in these communities and attempted to understand the many facets and rich variations of Aboriginal society. The authors, in their roles as anthropologists, natural scientists or health professionals, have studied various aspects of Aboriginal life. They have lived with their Aboriginal teachers, learning, puzzling and laughing with them, and sorrowing with them when relatives or friends have become sick or — too often — have died.

The diverse issues that underlie Aboriginal ill-health and health care are addressed in each of the three sections of this volume from a number of different perspectives. The first section, "Contemporary Crises in Health", outlines the nature of the health problems that burden Aboriginal communities and the socio-historical factors that have exacerbated them. In the second section, "Medicine and Health: The Traditional Systems", the authors describe some of the resources and the knowledge that Aborigines bring to the treatment of sickness, the theories that guide their diagnoses and interpretations, and the ecological correlates of good health. The final section, "Medical Strategies in Change", deals with the ways in which individuals perceive and adapt to changing health patterns and the pressures that influence their selection of indigenous or introduced medicines and procedures in times of sickness. Although the papers deal with diverse aspects of health and healing, they are linked by a common thread. Health, to Aborigines, is not a simple matter of good fortune, a prudent lifestyle or good diet. It is the outcome of a complex interplay between the individual, his territory of conception and his spiritual integrity: his body, his land and his spirit.

NOTES

[1] I am indebted to Dr Tom Gavranic, who first coined the analogy of an Australian invasion and kindly has given me permission to use the idea and to elaborate upon it in my own way.

[2] N. R. E. Fendall, "Auxiliaries and Primary Medical Care", *Bulletin of the New York Academy of Medicine* 48, no. 10 (1972): 1291–1300, at p. 1291.

[3] The report of the World Council of Churches, *Justice for Aboriginal Australians* (Sydney, 1981), provides a contemporary comment on these forces and the injustices suffered by Aborigines.

[4] M. Kamien, "Cultural Chasm and Chaos in the Health Care Services to Aborigines in Rural New South Wales", *Medical Journal of Australia* (Special Supplement) 2 (1975): 6–11.

[5] J. C. Reid, "Curing, Not Caring: Why Aboriginal Patients Abscond", *New Doctor* 8 (1978): 27–31; J. C. Reid, " 'Women's Business': Cultural Factors Affecting the Use of Family Planning Services in an Aboriginal Community", *Medical Journal of Australia* (Special Supplement) 1, no. 2 (1979): 1–4.

[6] The leading service in the training of Aboriginal health workers is the Northern Territory Department of Health. Although Aborigines had not, at the time of publication, achieved executive positions in the service, the health worker training and promotion structure allows the possibility that some may graduate to positions of authority.

[7] F. J. Bennett, "Primary Health Care and Developing Countries", *Social Science and Medicine* 13A (1979): 505–14, at p. 506.

[8] N. L. Radtke, "New Roles for Health Workers", *NFE Exchange* 15 (1979): 1–16.

[9] World Health Organization, *Report of the International Conference on Primary Health Care* (Geneva, 1978).

[10] Primarily the communities of central and northern Australia whose people follow, for the most part, their traditional ways, speak their own language, and have incorporated European technology and culture into their lives only to a limited extent.

Part One

Contemporary Crises in Health

If it used to be the case that the paucity of the data on Aboriginal ill-health enabled the wider Australian community to ignore this chronic tragedy, it is no longer so. During the 1970s, Health Departments throughout Australia improved their methods of collecting and recording demographic, mortality and morbidity statistics. The report on Aboriginal Health by the House of Representatives Standing Committee on Aboriginal Affairs (1979)[1] documented and deplored the health status of Aborigines and the lamentable public health facilities of their communities. The findings reported in the National Trachoma and Eye Health Program's Report (1980)[2] provide compelling evidence both of the high incidence of communicable and degenerative diseases among Aborigines and of their clear association with unsanitary and poorly serviced living environments.

The implications of statistics presented in official reports are often difficult to grasp. A more evocative description of the reality of the "Aboriginal health problem" is Moodie's[3] summary of the disease burden of a "not unusual" Aboriginal child admitted to hospital with "a small wardful of illnesses in the same body". The young patient is likely to be suffering from

> the presenting illness (say bronchopneumonia) + iron deficiency anaemia + roundworm and whipworm infestation + giardiasis + ringworm + pediculosis + diarrhoea + lactose intolerance + chronic suppurative otitis media + severe dental caries + a behavioural disturbance.

The medical conditions of the sick child pictured in this description are visible manifestations of a set of factors that plague many Aboriginal children from birth onwards and militate against escape from a pattern of debility and pain. This child very probably was born to a mother who already had several other young children, conceived within one or two years of each other. Unquestionably she would love them all, but her capacity to provide for their physical needs would be diminished by her own poor nutrition and chronic ill-health, by poverty and perhaps by family problems. Her emotional and financial resources might be strained by the drinking members of her family and by the hazardous environment of a crowded house lacking adequate toilets, piped water or any way of readily heating food or water. The severe stress of having to cope with these formidable social and economic disadvantages would be compounded by the anxiety of having to depend for her family's survival on European service agencies. Each time she must approach the European staff of the agencies, always in the role of supplicant, she may sense that they regard her as a less-than-competent human being. She would be an exceptional woman if she could retain her self-respect and dignity under such circumstances.

This section details selected aspects of the lifestyles and health of such individuals as the typical mother and child portrayed above. The chapters deal in turn with contemporary patterns of ill-health and their environmental correlates, the impact of contact on birth-rates and birth-spacing, the philosophy of child-rearing and child care of a central Australian community, and the social and historical context of petrol-sniffing in a desert community in southern Australia.

The first chapter, "A Fundamental Imbalance: Aboriginal Ill-health", is by Jack Waterford, a journalist who worked as a researcher with the National Trachoma and Eye Health Program and has been involved with Aboriginal community-based medical services. Waterford looks in detail at ill-health in Aboriginal communities throughout Australia and argues that the manifestations of ill-health reflect a fundamental disharmony between members of many Aboriginal communities and their physical, social and cultural environments.

Waterford points out that the disease pattern of contemporary Aboriginal society is similar to that of nineteenth-century Australia as a whole. The conditions that burden Aborigines today had ceased to be serious problems for the industrialized countries long before antibiotics were discovered or immunization campaigns introduced. Their decline was the result of improved nutrition, housing and public-health facilities. It is the *lack* of basic amenities, financial resources and nutritious foods in Aboriginal communities that places Aborigines, epidemiologically, one hundred years behind other Australians. To some extent, Waterford asserts, Western agencies could come to grips with infectious diseases without taking account of Aboriginal culture, lifestyle or values. But the threat of the future is posed by a second category of illnesses for which Western medicine has no answer. These are the "lifestyle" diseases such as diabetes and hypertension, associated with diet and exercise patterns, and secondary conditions such as alcoholism, drug abuse, trauma and mental illness. These problems can be tackled by Aborigines themselves, but only if they are given the resources and freedom to do so.

Gillian Cowlishaw's chapter, "Family Planning: A Post-contact Problem", provides an important synthesis of information on the determinants of Aboriginal fertility. Her paper dispels several myths about this issue. Some of the early — and not so early — commentators on Aboriginal society predicted that as birth-rates (for reasons unclear) dropped, its numbers would dwindle and the "race" die out. The issue was not how to plan for an Aboriginal future, but how most humanely to "smooth the dying pillow". The myth of the disappearing Aborigines persisted well into the 1950s and was current in popular belief until much later. In reality, Aborigines are having more children today than any other segment of the Australian population. Birth-rates (and, unfortunately, infant mortality rates) rival those of the populous developing nations. In many places, birth intervals are comparatively short, child-bearing begins at an early age and the completed family size is large. But demographic patterns were not always thus. It appears that prior to European colonization, birth spaces were long and births were infrequent. A range of factors, such as diet, prolonged breast-feeding and physiological processes acted as collective brakes on population growth. The change to a sedentary lifestyle, dietary shifts and other social and cultural adjustments to a new and imposed lifestyle have compromised the traditional checks on the birth-rate. For the grandmothers of many Aboriginal women living today, family planning was not a problem. Today, it is an issue of concern both to Aboriginal women and to health workers in their communities.

In the chapter "Child Health and Child Care in a Desert Community, 1970–1971", Annette Hamilton, who has studied Aboriginal child-rearing in central and northern Australia, looks at the way in which children are cared for in a remote desert community and how this care relates to child health. The impressions that other Australians hold of Aboriginal childhood are often contradictory. On the one hand, one often hears that Aboriginal parents love and indulge children and tolerate all manner of behaviour. On the other hand, the images of sickly, partially clothed, often runny-nosed Aboriginal children are often projected by the Australian media. Health personnel become frustrated as Aboriginal mothers bring their sick children again and again for care. The complex interactions of child-rearing patterns and environmental, historical and cultural variables are not well understood by researchers in this field, let alone by health personnel. Unaware of all the precursors of the recurrent diseases the children suffer, they sometimes blame the worried mothers for their children's plight. Yet the fact that mother and child are not causes, but victims, is becoming increasingly clear.

In her paper, Hamilton explains why "parental neglect" is a wholly inappropriate notion for understanding the health problems of Aboriginal children. The Aboriginal system of child-rearing rests on premises markedly different from those of the Western middle-class. Childhood morbidity has little to do with the actions, or inaction, of mothers. It is the outcome of a set of material and non-material factors which are the products of colonization and the pervasive changes it wrought in Aboriginal society.

The final chapter in this section, "Defiance or Despair?: Petrol-sniffing in an Aboriginal Community" by Maggie Brady and Rodney Morice, is a study of the social and historical matrix of one form of drug abuse in an Aboriginal community — petrol-sniffing. Unlike alcoholism, petrol-sniffing is confined to the young, and usually, but not always, to boys. Children learn to sniff from their peers at about eight or nine years of age and continue to sniff until mid- or late adolescence. Several initiatives to curtail sniffing in central and northern Australia have been tried. These include having the boys arrested for offences related to sniffing, sending them to outstations, providing recreational facilities or temporary adoption into the homes of relatives. None has been singularly effective; durable and widespread solutions seem a long way off. As with alcoholism, petrol-sniffing is not a cause but a consequence, and may be a barometer of the degree to which a community has lost purpose and self-respect.

Brady and Morice describe an applied research project being carried out at Yalata in South Australia. This study has focused on the juvenile offenders of the community and on the behaviours that are often labelled "delinquent" by the authorities. By working closely with the community and its council, and by relaying findings to the Aboriginal people concerned, the project is attempting to create an applied role for academic research. The paper shows dramatically how a web of controls has been spun round one small and displaced community by European agencies and describes their crippling effect on the Aborigines of the community. The issues discussed in this paper are complex and interdependent, but its message is clear: the hope for change lies at the level of community dynamics and particularly in a shift of authority and decision-making within the community from Europeans to Aborigines.

NOTES

[1] Australia. Parliament. House of Representatives Standing Committee on Aboriginal Affairs, ***Aboriginal Health*** (Canberra: Australian Government Publishing Service, 1979).

[2] ***National Trachoma and Eye Health Program: Report*** (Sydney: Royal Australian College of Ophthalmologists, 1980).

[3] P. M. Moodie, "Medical Aspects of Aboriginal Health", ***Australian Family Physician*** 6 (1977): 1309–17, at p. 1315. A detailed examination of the health of Northern Territory Aborigines in the late 1960s is found in Moodie, ***Aboriginal Health*** (Canberra: Australian National University Press, 1973). The literature available at that time is surveyed in ***The Health of Australian Aborigines: An Annotated Bibliography*** (Canberra: Australian Government Publishing Service, 1971).

1
A Fundamental Imbalance: Aboriginal Ill-health

Jack Waterford

INTRODUCTION

The poor health of Aboriginal Australians takes many forms, ranging from infectious disease of almost every kind to the lifestyle diseases associated with diet, exercise patterns, apathy and stress.

Some manifestations of this lack of health are discussed in this paper. But the argument of the paper is primarily that each of the conditions discussed is but part of a complex whole: reflecting a fundamental disharmony between members of many Aboriginal communities and their physical, social and cultural environments. This disharmony can be seen from many perspectives. The one used here is poor physical health, described and measured in Western scientific terms — but it could be described equally from any of a number of Aboriginal perspectives, as in several chapters in this volume.

The main purpose of this paper is to present some of the aspects of ill-health present in Aboriginal communities. In the final section are presented, briefly, some of the implications of this ill-health and what must be done about it. The single argument presented is that the whole complex of ill-health can be altered only by Aborigines themselves, and that the mechanism for achieving this alteration is the giving back to Aborigines of control over the factors that determine health: the whole living environment.

NOT AN UNRESEARCHED PROBLEM

By any standards, the health status of most Aboriginal Australians is appalling. This is in spite of a considerable investment of Western medical technology and trained manpower,[1] and, in recent years at least, an increasing attempt by those concerned with health care delivery to respond appropriately to the full range of needs of Aboriginal communities rather than with a curing approach to individual disease entities in individual cases. Health profiles for most Aboriginal Australians resemble more those to be found in the developing world than those that might be expected in a rich industrialized state.

There is no great need for further surveys, research or expeditions to discover and describe the health status of Aborigines in different areas. Already the medical and social sciences literature contains over 3000 references to aspects of Aboriginal ill-health, and innumerable inquiries into facets of the problem have been undertaken. More is probably known, in Western scientific terms, about the health status of the average Aboriginal Australian than of the average Caucasian Australian (Tatz, 1979).

In spite of this, the poor health persists. It will continue to do so until there is fundamental change in the life of Aboriginal Australians. And whatever change occurs will have to restore to Aboriginal communities and their members some harmony with their living environment: physical, social and cultural.

Of course, no community or individual is ever in complete harmony with the environment, and Aborigines suffered various forms of ill-health before European contact. But the coming of the Europeans fundamentally changed the picture of Aboriginal health – whether by the influence it had on the epidemiological dynamics of pre-existing disease entities (with the conversion of small, mobile groups of people into large, stationary ones, and changes in nutrition in particular), by the introduction of new infectious diseases (such as smallpox and syphilis), or by the introduction of living patterns that predisposed people to disease entities previously almost non-existent, but for which there was always a potential (such as diabetes, as a result of dietary changes, or hypertension, because of increased stress).

An example of the first change is middle-ear disease. The base of the chronic otitis media now observed in Aboriginal communities is the almost complete lack of appropriate health hardware – adequate and suitable housing, water supplies, nutrition systems and sewerage-disposal systems – which became a problem for large and stationary groups. This change converted a disease entity of probably moderate incidence but relatively short duration and few serious medium or long-term side-effects into a disease of high incidence, long duration[2] and often serious sequelae. This change is seen to effect in the experience of the Pintupi people, who "came in" out of the Western Desert to Papunya and other Central Australian communities in the 1960s, to face a holocaust of disease in which more than a quarter died. I have heard one Pintupi man refer to that period as "the time when the pus started coming out of the kids' ears".

An example of the second is smallpox, a disease unknown among Aborigines before European settlement, which probably killed ten times as many Aborigines during the nineteenth century as did settlers' bullets or poisons. Other examples are leprosy (probably introduced by Chinese, after European settlement), tuberculosis and many forms of sexually transmitted disease.[3]

The toll from the first two types of disease mentioned has, until recently, overshadowed other types of diseases that have arisen from the way in which Aborigines and their living patterns have been rearranged since white settlement: the so-called "lifestyle" diseases such as diabetes, hyperlipidaemia and hyperglycaemia. There of course has been no shortage of attention to secondary "lifestyle" entities such as apathy, alcoholism, trauma and mental disease, but more in the context of regarding them as "social" problems rather than medical ones. Both the primary and secondary lifestyle diseases are consequences of new Aboriginal living patterns: the former being more closely allied with diet and exercise patterns, radically altered by settlement and pauperization, the latter with the attack on the spirit that this has involved.

Before discussing some aspects of present Aboriginal ill-health, it is worth recording that Aborigines appear to be remarkably free of many of the hereditary or degenerative conditions, such as the cancers and nervous and sensory system disorders, that are a major form of morbidity among Europeans. Some of the degenerative conditions may never have come to the notice of Europeans because of the earlier toll from acquired conditions, but may become apparent as these conditions — usually more tractable — are dealt with. But the genetic isolation of pre-contact Aborigines, natural selection and their hunter-gatherer lifestyle may have given them a better potential for good health than their European counterparts. The significance of this is that the daunting Aboriginal health problems are usually acquired and usually tractable; the most daunting problems in Western society are frequently neither.[4]

INFECTIOUS DISEASE

Babies are born small for dates, possibly because of maternal malnutrition (averaging 2.8 kg in 1974) and have a high perinatal mortality. They are generally easily breast-fed and gain weight rapidly.

However, they have frequent chest infections during the first few months of life and it is not uncommon for these children to develop a perforated eardrum before they reach the age of six months. The

> children develop rapidly, but at some time between four and six months, their weight begins to fall off. Respiratory infections increase, with many children having repeated courses of antibiotics (averaging six courses a year each) for their chest and ear infections. Further problems such as scabies (60 per cent under the age of five are affected), parasitic infestation, bacterial enteric infections, and trachoma become more common after this age, the child being faced with a barrage of infections in a situation of poor nutrition. His poor nutritional state and recurrent illness often prevent his making good use of the food provided. During this first two years of life, he is likely to spend considerable time in hospital, much of this away from his family. There were 38 hospital admissions for the 18 infants studied in their first two years of life: only one had no time in hospital, the average stay was 12.5 weeks, with two children spending a total of a year in hospital and another three a total of six months each . . .
>
> As the child grows, he usually follows a growth curve below the normal, and continues to have repeated chest, throat, skin, gastrointestinal, eye and ear infections. This high infection rate does not encourage him to go to school regularly, and may lead to rheumatic heart disease, and glomerulonephritis from the repeated streptococcal infections . . .

The foregoing extract from a report on the development of Papunya children by Dr Trevor Cutter (1976) gives an all-too-familiar picture of growing up in an Aboriginal community, a picture that is still true of hundreds of communities throughout rural Australia, and even some urban communities. Thousands of Aboriginal children are being handicapped for life by an infectious barrage which begins soon after birth. The life of some, of course, is short, directly because of this infant disease: in 1979, one in every ten Aboriginal children was not living to the age of five (compared with one in forty non-Aboriginal Australians). Only ten years ago, twice as many children died before age five.

The infectious diseases flourish on living environments which permit a ready shedding and spreading of infectious organisms from one host to another: the persistence of the diseases and the damage they cause often are potentiated by run-down immunological systems, under a constant barrage from foreign protein — pathogens and ordinary organic matter — of all sorts. These hygiene diseases had largely disappeared among white Australians before the advent of antibiotics. It was economic development, bringing with it the health hardware previously mentioned, which modified the pattern of the diseases. Economic development has not yet reached many Aboriginal communities, particularly in the areas where these conditions are now most prevalent, the arid areas where many traditionally oriented communities live.

In such communities, Aborigines live in a "pool of infection": infectious secretions from one person are readily spread to others. Those who are most susceptible are those with least ability to make their escape from the reservoir — the children. Even when a person is "cured" by conventional Western therapy (usually antibiotics), he or she is quickly reinfected again. In such pools of infection, it is idle to single out single disease entities: those who are susceptible usually face a whole complex of infectious disease.

Table 1 below, drawn from National Trachoma and Eye Health Program findings, shows the prevalence pattern observed for three common infectious problems among rural Aboriginal communities throughout mainland Australia. Prevalence is very high in children under the age of two, it reaches its peak between the ages of two and three, and thereafter slowly declines, though remaining high in the pre-school and early school years. There were, however, wide variations between regions. For all that, the epidemiological pattern of peak prevalence in two- and three-year-olds was consistent in all areas. With nasal discharge, for instance, 78 per cent of the 2885 children under the age of ten seen in Central Australia were affected, whilst in the Torres Strait, the area of lowest prevalence, 20 per cent of children under the age of ten were affected. Similarly, trachoma prevalence was highest in the Central and Western Desert areas and lowest in the eastern and southern parts of the continent.

The National Trachoma Program did an intensive study of various environmental factors associated with such variations, considering a wide range of climatic variables — such as rainfall, humidity, evaporation, irradiation and exposure to sunlight — as well as a range of "hygiene factors" related to various forms of health hardware — housing, water supplies, waste and sewerage-disposal systems, and the range and quality of food available — possessed by different communities. This study showed that climatic factors were only secondary factors in disease prevalence: the most significant factor in determining disease was the community's store of health facilities.

Striking associations were found between disease prevalence and housing, as is shown in Table 2 below.[5] Similar associations were found between disease prevalence and such factors as:

(a) the way in which water supplies were arranged in the community: whether water for washing, cooking and laundry was available within or without dwellings, and whether there were adequate distribution points if inside dwellings (this study provided strong evidence against the ablution-block line of development);

Table 1. Patterns of Infectious Morbidity in Aborigines by Age

		% of Aborigines seen with condition		
Age	No. examined[a]	Follicular trachoma[b]	Nasal discharge	Otitis media[c]
0 - 1	2240	17.3	45.3	16.4
2 - 3	3182	34.4	58.2	19.8
4 - 5	4877	30.8	50.8	18.0
6 - 7	6453	23.9	40.3	16.0
8 - 9	5785	19.2	29.0	14.4
10 - 11	5400	15.6	17.3	13.0
12 - 13	4580	11.1	9.0	10.5
14 - 15	3639	6.9	4.0	10.6
16 - 17	2196	5.9	2.3	10.2
18 - 19	1690	5.1	2.4	9.0
20 +	21653	1.4	1.4	5.2
Total	61695	12.6	18.8	11.0

Source: National Trachoma and Eye Health Program, first screening survey of rural Australia.

Notes:

(a) The number of people examined varied slightly for each condition. For simplicity, the figure given is the number of people examined for follicular trachoma.

(b) Follicular trachoma is the first stage of trachoma, whereby follicles form underneath the eyelid and/or on the limbus of the eye itself. Eventually these follicles leave scars: a person with trachoma scars is said to have cicatricial trachoma. For cicatricial trachoma, there is a different prevalence pattern: briefly, the proportion of people with scars increases in each succeeding age group.

(c) Otitis media was defined as a wet or dry drum perforation, or "glue ear". Red drum was not included.

(b) waste-disposal systems: whether organic waste was adequately removed from the living environment;
(c) sewerage-disposal systems: whether sewerage was sufficiently removed from the living environment;
(d) the range and quality of food that was available.

Although discussion of infectious disease usually is concentrated on children, such diseases are by no means confined to the young. A range of conditions of their very nature primarily affect adults

Table 2. Infectious Morbidity in Aborigines According to Community Housing Status.

Range of Housing in Community	No. of Aborigines (All Ages) Living in Community		Disease Prevalence in Aborigines Under 20%			
	No.	% of sample	Follicular trachoma	Nasal discharge	Skin infection	Otitis media
1. All in community living in wiltjas[a]	2 895	4.8	46.8	54.1	10.3	10.8
2. Half of community in wiltjas, half in Stage 1 housing	5 325	8.8	36.3	49.3	7.3	6.9
3. All in Stage 1 housing, or half in wiltjas, half in unsatisfactory housing	18 233	30.0	27.4	37.8	7.4	6.8
4. Half in wiltjas, half in good housing, or half in Stage 1 housing and half in unsatisfactory houses (mostly latter)	11 852	19.5	17.5	27.3	6.0	4.4
5. Half in Stage 1 housing and half in good housing, or all in unsatisfactory houses	5 021	8.3	9.6	21.8	1.9	2.7
6. Half in unsatisfactory houses, half in good housing	12 908	21.2	5.8	21.8	2.1	2.4
7. All in good housing	4 552	7.5	4.3	13.0	3.3	2.0
All Categories	60 786		18.6	28.0	5.9	4.7
Equivalent Rate for Non-Aborigines	(31 219 under 20's)		0.9	1.2	0.6	1.1

Source: National Trachoma and Eye Health Program, first screening figures.

Note:

(a) Wiltja: a small, low dwelling, built at ground level to provide shelter and a wind-break. Traditional materials were leafy branches and other vegetation. Today, cloth, cardboard, corrugated-iron and other materials also are used.

(leprosy and syphilis are examples), while many adults endure lasting conditions greatly potentiated by the background of infectious disease they suffered as children. Some of these conditions are discussed below.

RESPIRATORY DISEASE

The body meets its environment particularly through its respiratory system, a large mucous membrane separating by only a few linings of tissue the body's most vital processes from the air and the physical environment. The level of respiratory disease is thus one of the most sensitive indicators of general health and the state of the environment. And, conversely, it is safe to predict the level of respiratory disease merely from an assessment of the physical environment.

Respiratory disease ranges from coughs, colds and "sniffles" to bronchitis, influenza and such lower respiratory tract conditions as pneumonia and emphysema. It also includes middle-ear disease, which stems in the main from the passage of infectious organisms from the respiratory tract to the middle ear via the eustachian tubes.

The high prevalence of respiratory disease in Aboriginal communities has been impressively documented,[6] but its ravages have been little checked. Respiratory disease is the most significant cause of mortality among Aborigines of all ages, and in terms of presentations to health workers, the most common and significant cause of morbidity.

Among children, the runny nose and the chronic cough can be almost universal. As well, in some settlements, up to half of the children at any one time will have discharging ears. These conditions set the pattern for long-term damage to the respiratory system, and to chronic conditions of adulthood.

Apart from the long-term sequelae of chronic respiratory disease complexes, there are significant short-term effects as well. One, of course, is discomfort. Others that should be mentioned are the hearing loss associated with discharging middle-ear infections (this most typically occurring in years of peak language and cognitive development) and the discrimination engendered by purulent discharges, whether from the ear, nose or other orifices. Of the former, it should be noted that the chronicity or repeated reinfection seen with Aboriginal otitis media may lead to long-term disadvantage: retarded development, accusations of inattention and laziness at school, and communication difficulties.

Many respiratory conditions are reasonably amenable to medical intervention, but the epidemiological patterns that have been observed suggest that treatment of affected individuals can at best only hope to check such conditions temporarily and reduce the damage they cause — and frequently cannot even do that. An attack on the pool of organisms associated with respiratory disease must involve a simultaneous treatment of all who are susceptible or potential hosts, along with measures designed to reduce the rate at which the organisms are shed and spread to other hosts: such public health measures as the reduction of crowding and the effecting of some separation of individuals from their living environments. These measures do not necessarily entail European patterns of socialization and housing: the development of the outstation or homelands movement, for example, may achieve some of the ends desired in terms of increasing personal space and cleaner environments.

NUTRITION, DEVELOPMENT AND GASTRO-INTESTINAL CONDITIONS

A host of studies have shown that members of Aboriginal communities have high levels of parasitic bowel infestations and enteropathogenic bacteria, associated with endemic diarrhoea, gastroenteritis, anaemia and the catch-all condition known as "failure to thrive". Other studies have shown reduced levels of vitamins and trace elements, including iron and zinc, in developing Aboriginal children and in their mothers.[7]

As with respiratory disease, the high prevalence of gastrointestinal conditions reflects high interpersonal physical contact and appalling living conditions, without health amenities. Nutritional deficiencies and their sequelae also are related to this environment, as they are to diet and to the use to which the body can put the type of food it consumes.

Anthropomorphic studies of developing Aboriginal children have indicated that many children develop at a slower rate than do their non-Aboriginal Australian cohorts, but would not do so given adequate nutrition and health care. The reduced development that does occur, usually in a complex of chronic infection, malnutrition and perhaps malabsorption, is associated with impaired intellectual development, which may retard the affected — even assuming they survive — for life.

The dietary status of members of many Aboriginal communities has been described by Jose and Welch (1970), and Ford and others

(1975) as protein–calorie malnutrition. Diet is heavily oriented towards carbohydrates, readily assimilable but poor in protein. Cereals that are consumed tend to be processed, and in their processing, to have lost much of their nutritional value. The "flour, sugar and tea", and ever-present "cool drink" (carbonated "soft" drinks), which is the basic dietary régime of so many communities, is a poor substitute for traditional "bush tucker", especially given changed exercise patterns, or for diets considered as normal or desirable in the wider Australian community.

Gastro-intestinal pathology and developmental impairment associated with poor nutrition cannot be considered in isolation: they are part of a whole complex of disease, mostly infectious or communicable, with which many Aboriginal children are affected. Each part of the complex plays its part: chronic respiratory or skin or eye disease taxes an already strained immunological system, which is thus the more at risk for other infections and nutritional impairment, which further tax the system, and so on.

With improving infant mortality rates, the persistence of high stillbirth and perinatal (first month of life) death-rates must be seen as being primarily due to low birth weights associated with poor maternal nutrition.[8] It is now well established that a mother's pre-pregnancy nutritional status is correlated with foetal development and early infant development (Naeye *et al.*, 1973).

SKIN INFECTIONS AND INFESTATIONS

Skin infections and infestations, including scabies, impetigo, tinea, lice and worm infestations, and infections associated with insect bites, wounds and ulcers are very prevalent in Aboriginal communities. Apart from the constant irritation, pain and inconvenience they cause (and their potential for engendering discrimination), there are long-term consequences, of which one of increasing concern is the close association between streptococcal skin infection, rheumatic valve conditions and kidney disease (Jose and Welch, 1969).

Skin conditions are largely environmental, with incidence affected primarily by the ease with which infectious material can pass between one host and another. Also significant in transmission dynamics are climatic factors, to an extent apparently greater than with most infectious diseases among Aborigines. Extremes of aridity and humidity predispose to skin disease. Thus the National Trachoma and Eye Health Program survey discovered that children in very humid tropical areas and in the very dry desert areas have higher prevalences of skin infections than children living in similar hygienic conditions but in more temperate climes.

Although rather more than a skin infection, leprosy can be considered under this heading. Leprosy was introduced in northern Australia, probably by Chinese or Macassans, late last century. By now, about 2000 Aborigines, more than 5 per cent of the Aboriginal population of these areas, bear the stigmata of the condition. Only about two in every hundred of these are considered infectious, although the numbers would be higher were many of the remainder not under constant drug therapy. In any event, although the incidence appears lower than was the case a decade or two ago, there are still no indications that the disease is under control.[9]

"SEXUALLY TRANSMITTED DISEASES"

This term is not wholly appropriate for Aboriginal communities. The inaptness arises because much such disease is asexually transmitted: these diseases are associated not only with sexual promiscuity but with a high physical contact environment, which permits the ready shedding and spreading of infectious organisms from one person to another.

The most commonly noted treponemal infections among Aboriginal communities are syphilis and gonorrhoea, but these may not be the most prevalent. The syphilis organism is closely related to the yaws organism and skilled venereologists have difficulty in distinguishing the two. Yaws probably was always endemic in Aboriginal society and may even have conferred some immunity to syphilis. Syphilis, an introduced disease, is increasing in incidence and prevalence in Aboriginal communities, while yaws, though commonly found serologically, appears to have almost disappeared as an active clinical entity. Perhaps 5 per cent of Aboriginal Australians, including one in ten of the sexually active (those aged fifteen to forty-nine), have syphilis, with a much higher prevalence in some areas. A further 5 per cent are serologically positive for either syphilis or yaws.[10] The upsurge in notifications in recent years indicates that secondary and tertiary syphilis conditions will appear in significant numbers in the next decade. What is more worrying is the increasing number of documented cases of asexually transmitted syphilis, in some cases in children from mere skin-to-skin contact in cold camping conditions.

Gonorrhoea, also introduced, is now also panendemic, and has been associated with reduced fertility among Aborigines until a generation ago. Incidence and prevalence as shown by such figures that are available appear to be fairly static, although still of substantial concern. One factor in keeping gonorrhoea under some control is perhaps the serendipitous effect on the gonorrhoea organism of the widespread use of systemic antibiotics in Aboriginal communities.

Almost completely undocumented is the existence of a wide range of urinary and genital tract conditions, which are probably even more common than syphilis and gonorrhoea. The organism associated with trachoma, *chlamydia*, is also associated with such urino-genital entities as non-specific urethritis, salpingitis and epididymitis: given the prevalence of trachoma, these might be expected to be widespread. Bacteriological studies, when undertaken, confirm a high prevalence of other pathogenic organisms in the genitals and urinary tracts of Aboriginal Australians.

However, there has been little research into the presence of such conditions in Aboriginal communities; such little research as has been done has been inhibited by culturally inappropriate case-finding techniques and technological difficulties (for example, the storage of specimens). Many Aboriginal men are not willing to be examined by a female nurse for any condition, let alone one in their genital regions. Similarly, there are considerable difficulties in conducting examinations of Aboriginal women, especially by male health staff. In some areas, blood-taking for serological examinations is said to be difficult for cultural reasons.

This does not mean that the high prevalence of such conditions has passed unnoticed or is not a subject of great concern in Aboriginal communities. One example of this concern was seen during the National Trachoma and Eye Health Program survey of the Pitjantjatjara communities. When the Program was meeting with the Pitjantjatjara council, to advise and plan with them a follow-up programme, they were asked by the council to provide a male doctor to examine for and treat venereal disease among Pitjantjatjara men. The council complained bitterly of the inappropriateness of nurse-based case-finding systems. One old *ngangkari* (Aboriginal healer) told the program's director, Professor Hollows, how the increasing incidence of genital infections was undermining the law (*Tjurkurpa*) and reducing the effectiveness of traditional healing practices; when he was a young man, the *ngangkari* said, he could deal with most complaints; now all the problems were "down there" (indicating genitals), and he could do nothing about them.

EYE DISEASE

Genetically, Aborigines appear more predisposed to good vision than Europeans. More Aboriginal children, adolescents and young adults have good vision as a proportion of their total numbers than do their non-Aboriginal counterparts, according to the National Trachoma and Eye Health Program survey, which covered about half of the rural Aboriginal population. Significantly, however, more older and elderly Aborigines are blind or suffer from visual handicaps than non-Aboriginal Australians of the same age. The survey showed that 19 per cent of Aborigines aged sixty or more who were seen were blind by legal "pension" standards; the figure for Europeans of the same ages is probably about one per cent (N.T.E.H.P. *Report*, 1980; Hollows, 1978b). Overall, fifteen in every thousand Aborigines seen were blind, but in some regions, particularly in the Central and Western Desert regions and in the cattle country of the Northern Territory and the Kimberley, the rates were much higher, running up to thirty-five per thousand. In the eastern and southern regions of Australia, blindness rates are lower and are closer to, but still exceed by a factor of two or three, the overall non-Aboriginal rate of about one per thousand.

An examination of the ocular pathology associated with blindness shows an immediate difference between Aboriginal and non-Aboriginal blindness. The conditions that blind Aborigines are not hereditary, nor, in the usual sense of the word, degenerative: most conditions are anterior segment disease, which either are treatable (and are thus avoidable) or which once should have been avoidable. By comparison, blindness among non-Aborigines seen is almost invariably caused by inherited or degenerative conditions, about which the current state of Western medical technology can do little.

International agencies concerned with the prevention of blindness have coined a phrase, "the overburden of avoidable blindness", to describe the proportion of people who can be saved from blindness by the effective combination of technology, skilled manpower and appropriate health care delivery systems. Using the criteria set by these experts, more than four out of every five Aboriginal blind persons are needlessly blind. There are probably 1500 blind Aborigines in Australia: 1200 of these would not have gone blind had they had available to them the blindness-preventing technology available to most white Australians.

Overall, about 3 per cent of Aborigines have significant avoidable visual handicaps. The bulk of this visual impairment comes from corneal disease, most of which is associated with damage caused by trachoma Trachoma is a disease of the conjunctiva (undersurface of the eyelids) and cornea (front of the eye). It begins, usually in childhood, with a form of chronic follicular conjunctivitis; the trachoma follicles recede in time, but leave in their wake scars and other changes to the cornea and eyelid. Initially, such changes may have little impact on vision, but in time they may progress to the point of collapse of the eyelid and marked ulceration of the cornea. Trachoma, by the damage it causes to the eyelid and front of the eye, also may rob the eye of much of its defence system against other infection and injury: eyes scarred by trachoma are more susceptible to other infections, while trauma to the eye (including surgery) is likely to have more serious effects in a trachomatous eye than in an unscarred one.

The follicular stage of trachoma is most apparent in childhood: particularly in arid areas, where virtually all Aboriginal children have or have had trachoma follicles. Overall, one in every three Aboriginal children seen by the National Trachoma Program had trachoma follicles, with a high prevalence in all but the eastern and southern regions of the continent. Two in every five Aborigines seen overall had some signs of trachoma, including two in every three Aborigines over the age of sixty. The epidemiological pattern of disease seen suggested that only in eastern and southern parts of the mainland is the disease under control and on the wane.

Among other eye conditions common in Aboriginal communities are lens disorders, mostly cataract, which is treatable if dealt with quickly enough, and a disease known as labrador keratopathy. Labrador keratopathy, the cattle industry's special contribution to Aboriginal eye health, appears to be caused primarily by exposure to ultra-violet irradiation and fine dust. It is rare in women and young men, and seems to be reserved for Aboriginal men who have worked with cattle for 20 years or more. Activity during the heat of the day, in highly dusty conditions, is probably the significant factor.

DENTAL DISEASE

Probably dental disease always has been endemic among Aborigines, but the incidence and severity of such disease has increased markedly because of profound changes in Aboriginal dietary patterns.

Few comprehensive surveys of Aboriginal dental health have been undertaken, although in some studies in western New South Wales, virtually all Aborigines surveyed had cavities, caries or gross gum inflammation or infection.[11] Many of these conditions could be improved by curative measures, but few Aborigines have access to dental services.

Many areas of Australia have low fluoride levels in natural water storages, and those who live in these areas are thus deprived of the protection by fluoride and other remineralizing agents against the development of caries. This deficiency is only partly being remedied by current water-supply programmes. The high carbohydrate intake, and a virtual absence of ordinary personal preventive measures — such as the use of toothbrushes — and the complete absence, or inadequacy, of dental services, makes serious and painful dental morbidity among Aborigines almost inevitable.

SOME DEMOGRAPHIC FACTORS

Before turning to the lifestyle diseases, it is appropriate to consider some demographic factors that affect income, reasonable expectations and the degree of stress that is to be encountered. These factors were perhaps best summarized by Professor Borrie, who said of Aborigines in his National Population Inquiry (1975) report:

> They probably have the highest growth rate, the highest birth rate, the worst health and housing, and the lowest educational, occupational, economic, social and legal status of any identifiable section of the Australian population.

Each of these factors plays an important role in health, just as health is an important factor affecting each of these characteristics.

The Australian Aboriginal population has a markedly different age structure from the rest of the Australian population. The number of children and adolescents, as a proportion of the population, is almost twice that to be found in non-Aboriginal communities, while the proportion of aged is about half. This has profound consequences for future population growth, but also has considerable immediate effects for the Aboriginal family. A typical Aboriginal family has twice as many dependents as a typical non-Aboriginal family.

For every Aborigine of working age (15–59 years) and capable of working, there are three others not of working age or not able to work. When present unemployment is taken into account, it is estimated (by the author, based on Australian Bureau of Statistics figures) that there is only one Aborigine currently drawing a wage for every eight Aborigines. By comparison, for non-Aborigines, there is approximately one adult wage-earner for each non-wage-earner. When education, skills and opportunities are taken into account, the wage the typical Aboriginal wage-earner receives may be half that of the typical non-Aboriginal wage-earner (Altman and Nieuwenhuysen, 1979).

These figures demonstrate the disadvantage that Aborigines suffer, and their dependency on social security and welfare payments. In fact, in many families, the major source of income is not wages or salaries, but pensions and child endowment, and, sometimes, unemployment benefits. Without such transfer income, average Aboriginal *per capita* income might be one half of that at present.

Acceptance of pensions and welfare assistance brings with it rules and regulations about living arrangements, and gives those who control the flow of such money extraordinary power over the lives of its recipients. The ensuing dependency and powerlessness has considerable consequences in terms of the stress encountered by members of Aboriginal communities, and in the way in which such stress is reflected in ill-health. The introduction of welfare benefits has not succeeded in widening opportunities for Aborigines: rather, it has served to impoverish them, and institutionalize their pauperization. At the same time, it has allowed outside agencies a more direct say in the way Aborigines organize their lives.

For Aborigines, this income and demographic situation means that there is little opportunity to save, to accumulate capital or to plan ahead. Life can revolve around the pension cheque schedule. One example of the implications of this can be seen with nutrition. The reality of the income situation is that there are few options about what food is purchased, even when there are opportunities for buying a wider range of food: it must be cheap, able to be spaced out, storable without refrigeration, or if not storable, readily consumed. The types of foods that meet these needs are tinned goods, processed cereals or "fast foods" and soft drinks. If vegetables and meat are bought, they can be purchased only for immediate use. Thus any alteration to dietary patterns involves far more than education about food qualities, about which most Aborigines are more knowledgeable than is generally assumed (as Meehan shows in her paper in this volume). Poor nutrition is primarily a consequence of present Aboriginal living conditions. Improvement in diet will follow increased income opportunities, or in some cases, the opportunity to move on to tracts of land that permit hunting and gathering, as is happening with the outstation movement.

With the present background of enforced dependency, new policies incorporating such slogans as "self-management" and "self-determination" have a hollow ring. What is needed rather than the present welfare system is a system that gives people some control over their lives and opportunities for independence. Among ideas advanced in this respect – which is not only a problem for Aborigines but also affects many poor non-Aboriginal Australians — are income maintenance schemes. Additionally, the development of land rights, the outstation movement, and Aboriginal corporate structures, may provide Aborigines with an economic base from which advancement is possible.

With these factors in mind, some of the "lifestyle" diseases and conditions are briefly considered.

PROBLEMS OF SETTLEMENT

Settlement living, with sedentary lifestyles and enforced idleness, and poor diet, together with low income and few expectations, interact together to produce a wide range of lifestyle diseases and conditions. The primary conditions are those such as diabetes, hypertension, hyperlipidaemia and hypocalcaemia, while secondary associated conditions include alcohol and drug abuse, mental illness and trauma. The conditions listed are but a fraction of the "lifestyle" disease that is present, but show the directions of major health problems of the future.

The statistical picture is rather more difficult to document, because research into Aboriginal ill-health has been primarily focused on infectious disease and its consequences. However, some figures are available.

In 1976, a Central Australian Aboriginal Congress survey, undertaken in conjunction with the National Trachoma and Eye Health Program, showed that, by urine analyis, about half of the several hundred Central Australian Aborigines surveyed were chemically diabetic. And in 1977, a Western Australian Department of Community Health audit of a Kimberley community showed that of 91 per cent of that population seen: 54 per cent of females and 67 per cent of males had low iron levels; 79 per cent of females and 86 per cent of males had low folate levels; 15 per cent of all seen were hypocalcaemic; 13 per cent were hypercholesterolaemic; 21 per cent were chemically diabetic; and 27 per cent were hypertensive (W.A. Community and Child Health Services, 1977). When it is considered that the last four conditions mentioned are conditions of adulthood, it can be seen that the true prevalence of these conditions among adult Aborigines in that community is about twice that given here.

Alcoholism in Aboriginal communities has been much noted and much deplored, and the subject of numerous inquiries.[12] Alcoholism is a major contributor to accident and injury. In New South Wales, where now a male Aborigine's life expectancy is about thirty-eight years (according to Dr John Ward, formerly director of the

Aboriginal health unit of the New South Wales Health Commission), alcohol can be expected to be associated with more than half of the deaths involved. Elsewhere, with life expectancy appearing to be about twenty years higher, alcohol is still a major factor in much mortality, and is associated with considerable morbidity, particularly in adults.

Other drug abuse, especially analgesic abuse, has been noted, particularly in less traditionally-oriented communities. Although the pattern of use is different, as with alcohol, a primary factor in abuse is an escape from the pressures, tensions and realities of ordinary community life. Drug abuse, including alcoholism, will not cease when people have wider opportunities and freer choices, but it certainly will be much reduced. At present, it must be seen primarily as a response to acute pressures and as an escape from the bleak reality that faces members of Aboriginal communities.

Mental illness in Aboriginal communities has been described frequently, notably by Cawte (1974) and Kamien (1978), although some feel that the norms against which abnormalities are noted are far from settled. Hollows (1978a) in particular has remarked how non-neurotic most Aborigines are, despite the most appalling disease, daily stresses and living conditions.

Eastwell (1978) identified much mental illness with "the stress of change", singling out the process of settlement in large numbers, role changes, pressure on family structures from new living arrangements and the stress on leaders of having to please both Aborigines and non-Aborigines simultaneously. Over a period of five years in the Northern Territory, he treated 435 people from a population of 10 500 people (5500 adults) with "head sickness", due to such problems as fear of sorcery (57 cases), depression (99 cases) and faints and turns (54 cases).

The stresses and tensions peculiar to Aboriginal communities also are reflected in the incidence of fights and accidents, and in the statistics for arrests and prison sentences. All indications are that these pressures will increase in the future.

Given that existing health care delivery systems so far manifestly have failed to alter greatly the pattern of infectious disease (which can, to some extent, be changed by regimentation and outside decision-making), it is difficult to see how Aborigines will be able to cope with this new crop of disease. In fact, only systems that embrace whole-hearted community involvement in decision-making, and which arise from the community, are likely to have any impact at all (Reid and Mununggurr, 1977; C.A.A.C., 1978).

IMPLICATIONS FOR HEALTH CARE POLICY

Health care delivery policies at present are highly ethnocentric, not only in their staffing and methodology but also in their assumptions about the choices that Aborigines may make. Because of this "cultural chasm" (Kamien, 1978), present health care delivery systems at best will remain only responsive to an environment endlessly churning out fresh victims and not a factor in their deliverance (Reid, 1979).

The World Health Organization counsels that health care planning should revolve around good health as a norm rather than focusing on ill-health in the development of policy and services. In Aboriginal communities, however, ill-health is the norm, and is an inevitable product of the way in which Aborigines, perforce, live. It is relatively easy for Western scientists to spell out the resources necessary to deal with many of the disease entities present, especially if temporary solutions or short-term relief from a particular disease is all that is sought. But given the way in which the situation of members of many Aboriginal communities determines and perpetuates disease, it is clear that outside technology is only a small part of the solution. The answers lie in real change to Aboriginal living situations, in creating a social, physical and cultural environment in which ill-health is only an occasional and remediable incident.

The conundrum was illustrated by a comment made to the author in 1978 by Frank Chulung, chairman of the Kimberley Land Council, who said: "The Government spends 98 per cent of its Aboriginal affairs money helping people deal with the problems they have because they have no land, and spends only 2 per cent acquiring land." The most hopeful sign, at present, is the development of community-based medical services, as part of an integrated plan for community development. Vague plans for "community participation" by official health authorities are no substitute for systems in which Aborigines plan, direct, implement and review the measures they need to take to produce good health. Equally, plans to increase numbers of Aboriginal health workers, a desirable aim in itself, will have no impact while health workers remain at the bottom of a Western-oriented health personnel hierarchy.

The most coherent objection to this development has come from Queensland and Western Australian Health Departments, whose arguments, as expressed for example by Mr Ray Young, Minister for Health in Western Australia (in 1979), are that Aboriginal medical services will involve duplication and will be too expensive. The reality is, that the present system could not be more expensive — yet it does nothing to resolve the problems that exist.

NOTES

1 Average direct expenditure on Aboriginal health by government — hospitals, health services and health staff — was at least $1200 per person per year in 1979. In the Northern Territory, only marginally the most extreme example, there was in 1979 a Health Department employee concerned with Aboriginal health for every twenty Aborigines: more than 75 per cent of such staff was non-Aboriginal. (Author's analysis based on federal and Northern Territory Health Department reports.) Kamien (1978) reports that Bourke in 1971 and 1972 — before the national explosion in health services — had sixty-six trained health care personnel, one of whom was Aboriginal, resident in the town, plus the services of visiting specialists, for an Aboriginal population of 700 and a European population of 3000.

2 The National Trachoma and Eye Health Program screened over 60 000 Aborigines — half of the rural Aboriginal population — and 40 000 non-Aborigines in all parts of rural Australia between 1976 and 1979. Screening was for eye disease, particularly trachoma, but some analysis of general health, including screening for middle-ear pathology, also was undertaken. Epidemiological analysis of the Program's findings for otitis media indicates that an eardrum perforation in a typical Aboriginal child persists for four years, on average, before healing over, whether being the one chronic condition or a series of closely following recurrent conditions. By contrast, analysis of the non-Aboriginal findings indicates that a non-Aboriginal case, itself considerably less common, heals over, on average, well inside two months (N.T.E.H.P. *Report*, 1980).

3 Moodie (1973), Hargrave and Jones (1980) and Abbie (1969) provide information and references on some of these introduced diseases.

4 See the National Trachoma and Eye Health Program *Report* (1980); and Abbie (1969) and Moodie (1973) about inherited and degenerative conditions generally.

5 The methodology and a fuller account of these environmental comparisons is to be found in the National Trachoma and Eye Health Program *Report* (1980). The author, who participated in the analysis of the Program's survey results, is anxious to avoid the use of the table presented as evidence that European housing is the answer to Aboriginal health problems. Housing development for Aborigines, in so far as it has occurred, has involved developments towards European-style housing, on the assumption that Aboriginal living and social patterns resembled or should resemble European ones. A house, for the purpose of the Trachoma Program analysis, was viewed as a convenient assemblage of health facilities, including:

(a) shelter from the heat and cold, wind and rain, and shade from the sun;
(b) adequate breathing space for all people using the house during the day and during the night;
(c) separation from the ground and pathogenic harbours;
(d) convenient access to water for washing, cooking and laundry;
(e) convenient space for storage and cooking of foodstuffs; and
(f) storage and security space in which belongings could be placed, secure from dogs, children and other adults.

How these facilities are assembled is an issue different from that of whether these facilities are to be available or not. If housing is to be an asset for health, the arrangement of its facilities must reflect the social realities and aspirations of those who are to use it: otherwise it will create more problems than it solves. See Heppell, 1979; N.T. Department of Health, 1979; and Australia. Parliament. Senate Standing Committee on the Environment, 1976.

6 The facts about the prevalence and nature of most of these conditions, particularly

for infectious diseases, are now generally well recognized, and no reference is made in the paper to the many studies that go to providing a national picture, unless for a particular reason. But see Moodie, 1973, 1977; Kamien, 1978; Gandevia, 1962; and Moran *et al.*, 1979.

[7] For instance, Moodie, 1973; Edwards, 1970; Gracey, 1973; and Harris *et al.*, 1970.

[8] Some mention also must be made of poor obstetrics, still a major factor in Aboriginal perinatal mortality. This problem is not merely one of remoteness, or poorly equipped health service facilities, since it occurs at some of the best-equipped hospitals.

[9] See Hargrave and Jones, 1980; and annual reports of Northern Territory and Western Australian Health Departments.

[10] This is the author's assessment, based on state and Northern Territory community screenings. See Department of Health (N.T. Division) reports; and Jorgensen, 1978; and Garner *et al.*, 1972.

[11] Health Commission of New South Wales, 1978; and Kamien, 1978.

[12] See Australia. Parliament. House of Representatives Standing Committee on Aboriginal Affairs reports, 1977 and 1979.

REFERENCES

Abbie, A. A., 1969. *The Original Australians* (London : Muller).

Altman, J. C., and Nieuwenhuysen, J., 1979. *The Economic Status of Australian Aborigines* (Cambridge : Cambridge University Press).

Australia. Parliament. House of Representatives Standing Committee on Aboriginal Affairs, 1977. *Alcohol Problems of Aboriginals* (Canberra : Australian Government Publishing Service).

——, 1979. *Aboriginal Health* (Canberra : Australian Government Publishing Service).

——. Senate Standing Committee on the Social Environment, 1976. *The Environmental Conditions of Aborigines and Torres Strait Islanders and the Preservation of Their Sacred Sites* (Canberra : Australian Government Publishing Service).

Cawte, J. E., 1974. *Medicine is the Law* (Honolulu : University Press of Hawaii).

Central Australian Aboriginal Congress. House of Representatives Standing Committee on Aboriginal Affairs, 1978. Transcript of Evidence, vol. 3 : 1511–1619, 26 June; vol. 7 : 4120–26, 2 November, *Hansard* (Canberra : Australian Government Publishing Service).

Commonwealth Department of Health, Northern Territory Division, 1978. *Annual Report 1977–78* (Canberra : Australian Government Publishing Service).

Cutter, T., 1976. "An Environmental Approach to Health at Papunya", unpublished ms. (Alice Springs : Central Australian Aboriginal Congress).

Eastwell, H. D., 1978. "The Mental Health Movement : Part 1. The Stress of Change", *Aboriginal Health Worker* 2, no. 3 : 4–9; Part 2 : 2, no. 4 : 8–11.

Edwards, L., 1970. "Malnutrition and Disease in Pre-school Aboriginal Children in the Walgett Area of N.S.W.", *Medical Journal of Australia* 2 : 1007–12.

Ford, G., Jakeman, M., Jose, D., Vorbach, E., and Kirke, D., 1975. "Migration Inhibitory Factor Production by Lymphoid Cells of Australian Aboriginal Children with Moderate Protein-Calorie Malnutrition", *Australian Paediatrics Journal* 11 : 160–64.

Gandevia, B., 1962. "The Prevalence of Signs of Chronic Respiratory Disease in Pintubi and Walbiri Aborigines at Papunya, Central Australia and Warburton, Western Australia", *Medical Journal of Australia* 2 : 237–42.

Garner, M., Backhouse, J., Moodie, P., and Tibbs, G., 1972. "Treponemal Infection in the Australian Northern Territory Aborigines", *Bulletin World Health Organization* 46 : 285–93.

Gracey, M., 1973. "Enteric Disease in Young Australian Aborigines", *Australia New Zealand Journal of Medicine* 3 : 576–79.

Hargrave, J. C., and Jones, E. R., 1980. *Leprosy in Tropical Australia: A Short Guide for Field Staff in the Diagnosis, Treatment and Management of Leprosy* (Darwin : N.T. Medical Service).

Harris, M., Duffy, B., and Beveridge, J., 1970. "Studies on the Small Bowel of a Group of New South Wales Aboriginal Children", *Medical Journal of Australia* 1 : 356–59.

Health Commission of New South Wales (Aboriginal Health Section, Dr J. Ward), 1978. House of Representatives Standing Committee on Aboriginal Affairs, Transcript of Evidence, vol. 1 : 389–453, 19 April, *Hansard* (Canberra : Australian Government Publishing Service).

Heppell, M. (ed.), 1979. *A Black Reality* (Canberra : Australian Institute of Aboriginal Studies).

Hetzel, B., Dobbin, M., Lippman, L., and Eggleston, E. (eds.), 1974. *Better Health for Aborigines?*, Report of a National Seminar at Monash University (St Lucia : University of Queensland Press).

Hollows, F., 1978a. "Aboriginal Eye Health and What Must be Done".

———, 1978b. "The Ocular Status of Old Aborigines", unpublished mss. (Sydney : Department of Ophthalmology, University of New South Wales, and National Trachoma and Eye Health Program).

Jorgensen, D., 1978. House of Representatives Standing Committee on Aboriginal Affairs. Transcripts of Evidence, vol. 5 : 2962–98, 2 August, *Hansard* (Canberra : Australian Government Publishing Service).

Jose, D. S., and Welch, J. S., 1969. "Studies of Australian Aboriginal Children : Streptococcal Infection, Heart Reactive Antibody and Subclinical Rheumatic Carditis", *Australian Paediatrics Journal* 5, no. 4 : 209–18.

——— and ———, 1970. "Growth Retardation, Anaemia and Infection, with Malabsorption and Infestation of the Bowel: The Syndrome of Protein-Calorie Malnutrition in Australian Aboriginal Children", *Medical Journal of Australia* 1 : 349–56.

Kamien, M., 1978. *The Dark People of Bourke* (Canberra : Australian Institute of Aboriginal Studies).

Moodie, P. M., 1973. *Aboriginal Health*, Aborigines in Australian Society 9 (Canberra : Australian National University Press).

———, 1977. "Medical Aspects of Aboriginal Health", *Australian Family Physician* 6 : 1309–17.

Moran, D., Waterford, J., Hollows, F., and Jones, D., 1979. "Ear Disease in Rural Australia", *Medical Journal of Australia* 2 : 210–12.

Naeye, R., Blanc, W., and Paul, C., 1973. "Effects of Maternal Nutrition on the Human Fetus", *Paediatrics* 52, no. 4 : 494–503.

National Population Inquiry : Population and Australia, 1975. (Canberra : Australian Government Publishing Service); and *Supplementary Report*, 1978.

National Trachoma and Eye Health Program : Report, 1980. (Sydney : Royal Australian College of Ophthalmologists).

Northern Territory Department of Health, 1979. *An Environmental Survey of Aboriginal Communities 1977–78* (Darwin : Government Printer).

Reid, J. C., 1979. "Aboriginal Health in the 1970's and 1980's", *Cumberland College Reports*, no. 16 (Sydney).

——, and Mununggurr, D., 1977. "We are Losing our Brothers: Sorcery and Alcohol in an Aboriginal Community", *Medical Journal of Australia* (Special Supplement) 2 : 1–5.

Tatz, C., 1979. *Race Politics in Australia* (Armidale : University of New England).

Western Australia. Community and Child Health Services, 1977. *Annual Report* (Perth : Government Printer).

2
Family Planning: A Post-contact Problem

Gillian Cowlishaw

INTRODUCTION

The rate of infant mortality among Australian Aborigines today is excessively high when compared with that of other Australians. In some districts, it can be up to ten times higher than the overall Australian rate of approximately 20 deaths per 1000 live births. The rate of deaths in 1–4-year-olds is even higher in comparison with the overall rate. Another and related problem, of which Aboriginal women complain, is the dramatic increase in the frequency of births. Older women say that they did not conceive as often "before", and consider it quite wrong for a child under at least four years to be displaced by another infant. Even the first stages of pregnancy are seen as a threat to the health of a breast-feeding child. These findings, from the author's work among Rambarnga women at Goinjimbi in southern Arnhem Land, have been confirmed in other areas (e.g. Reid & Gurruwiwi, 1979). The intensity of customary nurturance patterns and the indulgence of young children among Aborigines seem to demand few and well-spaced births. A study of traditional reproductive patterns among Aborigines is thus of importance if we are to understand the health problems of Aboriginal children. These are not simply the result of particular contemporary conditions and cannot be solved by purely medical procedures. The reason for the low traditional birth-rate is not well understood, but is of general medical and anthropological interest.

There are two common misconceptions, which this paper hopes to correct. The first is that Aboriginal women always and everywhere suffered from a high and constant level of fecundity. The second is that traditional Aboriginal society was egalitarian. The positive side of these views is as follows. Firstly, evidence will be given that Aboriginal fertility was low in the traditional situation. The sudden increase in birth-rates since European contact has caused and is causing severe stress. It is important for health workers and Aborigines to understand the reasons for this increase and appreciate the Aboriginal women's view of the burdens that result. Secondly, it will be shown that social relations are as important in determining fertility levels as are directly physiological considerations. As with any other society, there were, in Aboriginal groups, conflicts of interest between categories of people, and while the interests of one section were protected by social structures, the others had to pursue their own interests as best they could. In particular, Aboriginal society was geared to the interests of older men. Though women had a good deal of autonomy, pursuit of their own interests was often at the expense of their duties to men.

Fertility is a term used in two distinct ways, and we shall be dealing with both. Firstly, it is a demographic concept, referring to the birth-rates in populations. The first part of this paper is demographic, consisting of an assessment of the fertility levels of Aboriginal women prior to European contact. But fertility also is used in the medical sense, to refer to a woman's ability to conceive. This could be described as physiological fertility, which is obviously a major factor determining population fertility. The remainder of the paper will attempt to account for the low population fertility, as described below, in terms of physiological fertility.

As a basis for identifying a low birth-rate, this paper uses the same measure of population fertility as employed by Nag (1962 : 15–16) in his survey of fertility among populations studied by anthropologists, where no modern contraceptives are used. The two statistics are total maternity ratio (live births per woman, considering women over age 45) and maternity ratio (live births per women, considering all women).

FERTILITY OF THE PRE-CONTACT ABORIGINAL POPULATIONS

There is a paucity of data on pre-contact Aboriginal populations. From the available data collected, it seems that Aboriginal birth-rates were even lower than those of the !Kung of Africa, who also had unexplained low fertility (Howell, 1976 : 147). Here a very brief summary of this data will be presented, giving a total maternity ratio, maternity ratio and sterility rate. (See Table 3 below.) As none of the observers was a demographer, there are problems with the material. Notes on the manner of collection and the degree of contact the population had experienced are available (Cowlishaw, 1979). In all, the rates are very low. Though some writers have attributed this low birth-rate to post-contact trauma, the areas with least contact show the same low rates, and there is no evidence that birth-rates decreased with contact. Even if some decrease occurred, it seems probable that it was from an already low rate.

Other observations of frequent sterility and a low birth-rate were made by Spencer and Gillen (1968 : 52n), Hernandez (1941 : 123–24) and R. M. and C. H. Berndt (1943 : 247, 275).

Table 3. Summary of Historical Data on Aboriginal Maternity Ratios

Date Collected	Collected by	Maternity Ratio	Total Maternity Ratio	No. Childless (%)
1971 (from historical documents)	Barwick, 1971		1.5 to 2.0	20.0
1849–1922 (originals)	Krzywicki, 1934		4.6 to 5.0 3.8 to 4.3 (amended)	
1899	Roth, 1908	2.3		15.0
1900	Roth, 1908	1.4		16.0
1933	Sharp, 1940	2.1 2.1		21.7 22.0
1943	Berndts, 1943		3.0 (approx.)	
1948	Billington, 1960	2.8 3.0 1.8		
1962	Long (in Peterson, 1972 : 158)	2.1		25.0
1960	Hiatt, 1978		2.5 3.3	16.0[a] 8.0[a]
1967	Peterson, 1972	1.6		36.0
1975	Hiatt, 1978		4.3	0.0
1962 (from public documents)	Jones, 1963		4.3	16.5[b] 31.5[c]
Comparisons:				
! Kung	Howell, 1976	3	4.7	16.0
	Nag, 1962			
	Highest	5.6	10.4	
	Median	3.2	5.8	
	Lowest	1.7	2.6	
White Australians	(Llewellyn-Jones, 1972 : 82)			6.5

Notes:

The material is summarized in order of the date it was collected. (Barwick uses early sources.) This does not necessarily represent the degree of contact, which varies from district to district. For detailed assessment of these sources, see Cowlishaw, 1979.

(a) Total sterility ratio; (b) North Division; (c) Northern Territory.

Contrary to the view of Rose (1968 : 203), who asserted that Aboriginal women who lived to menopause had at least eighteen children, the evidence supports the view that the average number of children borne by a woman was about four.

It might be objected that the nature of this data does not allow us to distinguish between a low birth-rate and high infant mortality. Might not the birth-rate and the infant mortality rate always have been as high as they are today? There is evidence that this is most unlikely. Firstly, possible reasons for a high rate of infant mortality in the past have not been demonstrated. The causes of the current high infant mortality rate are such diseases as pneumonia, gastroenteritis and dysentery, which are generally the result of unhygienic conditions in sedentary camps (Jones, 1963 : 47–51). These are post-contact phenomena associated with settlements and missions, and the associated crowding, poverty and lack of hygiene. Such conditions are not characteristic of traditional Aboriginal nomadism. Secondly, with some exceptions, the ethnographic literature does not include observations of a high infant mortality rate in nomadic conditions.

There is also direct evidence that infant mortality has increased rather than decreased. While infanticide may have been reduced (though this would be difficult to ascertain), and medical intervention certainly would have saved the lives of some infants, infant deaths outstrip these reductions by a wide margin (Jones, 1963 : 47, 53–4). That is, both the birth-rate and infant mortality have increased sharply in settlements, missions and station camps.

Thirdly, and most important, Aboriginal women repeatedly report that they are conceiving more often than previously (White, 1977 : 278; Reid & Gurruwiwi, 1979). Attitudes to the current birth-rate confirm the view that early pregnancies and short birth intervals are new phenomena. This sharply increased birth-rate has upset women's traditional nurturance patterns and is not conducive to the good health of infants. In fact, the level of indulgence of children among Aborigines hardly could be customary unless the numbers of children were low.

In the following sections, the factors that could account for the low physiological fertility that seems to have characterized traditional Aboriginal populations will be examined. These will be dealt with under the headings of the probabilities of ovulation, of conception and of parturition. In conclusion, the ramifications of changed fertility patterns for maternal and infant health and medical services in Aboriginal communities will be discussed.

FACTORS AFFECTING OVULATION

Before taking up the question of reduced probability of ovulation, it is of interest to note that several observers have commented that Aboriginal women menstruate infrequently or irregularly (Abbie, 1960 : 142; Roheim, 1933 : 233; Hamilton, pers. comm.). Infrequent and irregular menstruation is prima facie evidence that ovulation is infrequent and irregular. Evidence of factors that would affect ovulation are examined below, under the headings: nutrition and energy expenditure, lactation and fallopian tube blockage.

Nutrition and Energy Expenditure

It has been convincingly shown that today, European girls reach menarche 2½ to 3½ years earlier than they did a century ago. This trend correlates with that of height and weight, indicating that better nutrition may be the major cause (Tanner, 1968 : 25–27). Experimental evidence that a relationship between body weight and ovulation exists is set out by Frisch and McArthur (1974). They show that a certain level of stored, easily mobilized energy is necessary for menstrual cycles to occur. They have found that undernutrition causes a delay in the adolescent growth spurt that normally precedes menarche, and that menarche also is delayed. Undernutrition also can lead to cessation of previously established menstrual cycles. Frisch (1978 : 22) also has provided historical evidence that nutrition has a direct effect on reproductive ability. That is, an undernourished woman has not only a lower probability of ovulating and thus of conceiving but also has a higher probability of a miscarriage or a stillbirth and her lactational amenorrhoea lasts longer.

There is evidence that the body fat of both !Kung Bushmen and Australian Aborigines was very low in pre-contact populations, and this factor may be responsible for the low fertility in both groups. Measurements of the weight for height and age of Aborigines with minimal contact with European foods showed them to be considerably leaner than their white counterparts. Apart from the contrast between blacks and whites, there is a marked contrast between male and female Aborigines. There is a decrease in weight with age after early adult life, and this is more marked in women (Billington, 1960 : 31).

The only works available giving details of food consumption are those of McCarthy and McArthur (1960) and Meehan (1975); both of these studies are from Arnhem Land. The general conclusions drawn from these and other studies of a more general kind are that in such an environment, the staple dietary needs of the people are adequately supplied by only a few hours of work a day.

It is clear from Meehan's study that the collection of food, particularly the staple shellfish, which was collected mostly by the women, did not require their maximum effort. But, of course, flour was used regularly at the time of this investigation. Meehan (1975 : A44) calculated how much vegetable matter would have been equivalent to the amount of flour used and concluded that the women could have gathered sufficient yams. She considers that "a small change in the population structure, an increase in the yam yield, a lowering of the calorific intake — or better still a combination of all three, renders the task feasible." But it must be pointed out that the population may have been unbalanced in any one of a number of ways, with perhaps fewer women and more men, old people and children. In such a situation, the women may have suffered considerable strain on their energy resources. The strenuous task of yam collection also would require an extra calorie intake by women, to maintain the same nutritional level.

There is solid evidence that the women of Arnhem Land provide more food and receive less. As the women bring food in every day, the family is primarily dependent on their efforts. Women sometimes go without to provide for their children (Meehan, 1975 : 211). Men have control over the distribution of meat and generally consume more of it. Where women are forbidden to eat kangaroo, the men may choose (or not) to lift the taboo (McCarthy and McArthur, 1960 : 156). When men are involved in the large ceremonies, women provide staple foods for them. Men do not provide food for women's ceremonies. Peterson (1972 : 118) points out that men contribute no vegetable food to the collective diet, but women do contribute meat, and this meat sometimes provides the bulk of the meat in the diet. Women are regular providers of food from childhood to old age. Men hunt intermittently for a shorter part of their life-span.

Actual consumption patterns also can be relevant here. The author's own observations among the Rambarnga indicate that the men's habit of eating large quantities of meat contrasts markedly with the women's and children's delicacy and control, and frequent self-sacrifice. A fastidiousness bordering on disdain for food is often displayed. The shaming of children, especially young girls, who show greed provides the explanation for the development of such attitudes. There is evidence that "nutritional imprinting" occurs, so that nourishment patterns formed early in life are not easily altered later (Fomon, 1967 : 271–72).

The gorging of meat by men also contrasts with women's behaviour, in that women's food taboos most frequently apply to the larger animals and fish, so that it is usually only men who can indulge themselves in this way. At Goinjimbi, all the young women were observed to be restricted in their choice of food at some time because of some taboo. For instance, a husband and father sat down in front of a whole roast bush turkey on one occasion, while his wife and daughters chewed damper. This was because a classificatory kinsman, often resident at another community, was undergoing his initiation, and during many months this fact placed a dietary restriction on his "mothers" and "sisters". Most of the young girls' restrictions are intended to improve the efficacy of the initiation rites of one or another real or classificatory male relative. As buffalo meat is available at Goinjimbi and is not the subject of taboos, these girls and women do not suffer deprivation today, but evidence of the extent of the taboos on the major sources of protein indicate possible deprivation in the past, most markedly for young girls and pregnant and lactating women. Kaberry (1939 : 214) says that female relatives are most endangered by death, so that they must observe a taboo on meat and their diet is mainly limited to vegetable foods, small fish, snakes and witchetty-grubs.

Kaberry (1939 : 100) writes that girls also suffer food restrictions at puberty:

> At her first menses the girl goes apart with her mother, away from the men and young children. She must not eat certain foods — porcupine, long-necked turtle, emu, native companion, little kangaroo, dog, opossum, snake, turkey, iguana, barramundi and wild-cat. . . . Since all meat caught by the men is *gunbu*, taboo, it follows that her diet is practically restricted to vegetable foods, fruits, and small fish procured by the women.

Most other accounts of food taboos indicate similar restrictions on the major sources of protein for girls and women.

Medical evidence that such taboos can cause a major nutritional handicap comes from a contemporary observer who found that mourning taboos caused serious malnourishment in the south-west Kimberley region of Western Australia (Ackerman, 1975 : 124). This is evidence that while women may have access to food, they still could suffer severe physiological consequences because of cultural proscriptions. Thus simple availability of food is not the only issue. Women may have been undernourished "voluntarily", due to food taboos, the demands of others, training in childhood to eat little and the overriding claims of their dependent males.

It could be argued that as the women eat what they wish when out collecting, they are unlikely to suffer shortage of food. But it must be remembered that they may be punished and shamed if they continually supply insufficient food. Thus young girls refrain from eating large fish and are encouraged to bring such creatures home for their fathers. The women can eat only a limited amount when out gathering. Also some of the traditional staples require preparation. If they are not to be considered greedy, women will divide what they collect, and in balancing the immediate satisfaction of eating against the satisfaction of fulfilling obligations, make a compromise.

The argument so far consists of the following points: Lack of body fat in women causes anovulation, probably due to insufficient energy reserves. Aborigines were lean, and the women were significantly leaner than the men. This was so partly because of differential rights to some foods and partly because of greater energy expenditure. Pre-contact Aboriginal fertility was low.

Fertility has increased markedly on missions and government reserves, where flour and sugar are provided. The significant factors leading to this increased fertility would seem to be a greatly reduced energy expenditure on the part of the women and an increased carbohydrate intake, leading to a build-up of body weight.[1]

Lactation

It is the contraceptive significance of lactation rather than that of nutrition that usually has been considered the major reason for long birth intervals among hunter-gatherers. This contraceptive effect is due to the production of prolactin, which is the hormone responsible for the cessation of ovulation. Prolactin production is stimulated by suckling and it is present immediately after suckling in the first three months after birth, at levels equal to those obtained during the last phases of pregnancy, when prolactin is at its highest level. The level falls fairly rapidly by half during the first hour after suckling, but the basal level remains high for three months after a birth, gradually declining over the following months. Thus the time elapsing after a birth seems to be one independent factor in reducing the level of prolactin (Delvoye *et al.* 1976; Healy & Burger, 1977).

It has been argued that, when infants depend exclusively on breast milk for a number of years because no sufficiently soft supplementary food is available in the environment, the level of lactation will be sufficiently high to inhibit ovulation. It was alternative food sources for infants that released human fertility from this control that existed among hunter-gatherers. Another aspect of this view is the frequency of suckling. Serum prolactin levels fall swiftly after suckling ceases, but among hunter-gatherers, where babies are virtually continuously suckled for a number of years, there will be a sufficiently continuous high level of prolactin to block ovulation. Non-nutritive suckling is common where the breast is used as a pacifier among hunter-gatherers. By contrast, among primitive agriculturalists, babies commonly are left in the village during the day while the mother works in the field. Breast-feeding has been limited during most of European recorded history. The modern four-hour feeding schedules mean periods of some hours between feeds, and longer during the night. Thus the "natural" physiological process, which both provided nutrition for infants and ensured that the mother did not conceive again, has ceased to be effective in all but hunter-gatherer populations.

There are several problems with these arguments. The major weakness is the use of the suckling factor to explain a four-year birth interval, without attention to changes in the lactation or suckling pattern over this period. Infants gain a progressively smaller proportion of their nutritional needs from breast milk. Studies of women of the New Guinea highlands show that each year the milk supply is progressively reduced, from 700–400ml in the first year, to 400–200 ml in the second and around 200 ml thereafter, until weaning (Bailey, 1965 : 36). The quality of the milk is somewhat improved in both protein and solids content until the fourth year, but not nearly enough to counteract the lessened quantity, let alone the increasing nutritional needs of the child (Becroft, 1967 : 600). Bailey (1965 : 47) concludes her study of breast-feeding in New Guinea with the observation that there is no evidence of a correlation between quantity of milk consumed and the growth of the infants beyond 6–12 months. Thus the level of lactation is reduced independently of the provision of supplementary foods.

Non-nutritive suckling reduces in frequency with age. From the author's observations, many Aboriginal infants over a year old only suckle occasionally during the day, and seldom at night. Both decreased total suckling time and increased length of time between feeds will occur as a result of the infant's increased mobility, and emotional independence, and also because of the reduction in the amount of milk available.

A second point is that Aboriginal infants from the age of six months are given almost anything to eat that they ask for. McArthur (1960 : 123) described the range of foods Arnhem Land infants were given from six months of age and says that by the age of about two years, solid foods form the bulk of the diet. One-year-olds can eat several adult foods and gain a good deal of nourishment from them. These children certainly continue to suckle, but it cannot be asserted that they are required to depend on breast milk because of the lack of grain foods to supplement the diet. Supplementary foods are *necessary* after six months. Thus re-establishment of ovulation can be expected as a function of the time elapsing since parturition.[2]

Finally, the increase in birth rates that has occurred on missions and government stations is not preceded by a reduction in suckling. If anything, the sedentary life, with no necessity to collect food, means that infants have more access to the breast and, from observations made at Goinjimbi, take advantage of this fact. The availability of supplementary food has not been shown to reduce suckling time.

Fallopian Tube Blockage

In some parts of Australia, Aboriginal girls underwent an introcision operation at puberty. There are two ways in which such an operation could have an effect on fertility. The first is by some direct physical damage to the reproductive organs, which is unlikely. The other possible effect is through infection, causing infertility by a blockage of the fallopian tubes. Expert opinion is that such an effect is unlikely also. Sterility also is observed to exist in areas where there is no such initiation for girls, and this precludes it as a general explanation.

The syndrome of "one child infertility" that has been identified in "Western" populations also must have occurred among Australian Aborigines. The condition referred to is fallopian blockage, which occurs because of infection at parturition. This would be at least equally likely to occur among Aboriginal women. Perhaps more significantly, fallopian blockage is even more likely to occur as the result of procured or spontaneous abortion. In all societies, women have known how to procure abortions by one of a number of methods. Aborigines are no exception. When girls conceived early or when a woman conceived when she still was breast-feeding, abortion could be a solution to the problem. It is likely that such girls and women were the most naturally fertile. Thus a proportion of the 20 per cent of women who had no offspring may have suffered oviduct blockage as the result of aborting an infant when young.

FACTORS AFFECTING CONCEPTION

The two factors that seem to be of importance here are coital frequency and male fertility. When demographers suggest that the age at marriage and the delay of widow remarriage are important determinants of birth rates, they really are referring to frequency of sexual intercourse. Aboriginal girls generally marry at or before puberty, and when they marry later, there are few controls on premarital sexual activity. Thus marital status is not a useful variable.

Frequency of Sexual Intercourse

Frequency of intercourse as a factor affecting the fertility of a population has been discussed by Nag (1972). He points out that if intercourse commonly occurs less than four times a week, the chances of conception are significantly decreased. Now it may be argued that such a consideration would have no relevance to the Australian Aborigines, since there are virtually no single women. In general, girls marry young and widows remarry quickly. This question requires further examination. It is possible, for example, that older women sometimes are rejected by husbands who have new young wives. Secondly, the opportunity for intercourse may not arise, either because some women deliberately subvert the sexual wishes of their possible partners[3] or because the couple cannot achieve sufficient privacy. Thirdly, there is the existence of post-partum sex taboos. The divergent opinions that have been expressed about permissiveness among Aborigines are not surprising (e.g. Berndt and Berndt, 1964 : 159; Tonkinson, 1978 : 82–83; Stanner, 1933 : 27). They indicate the difficulties of observation in the area of sexuality. But while the rules and restrictions placed on sexual expression differ from society to society, everywhere these rules are the subject of intense feeling and powerful sanctions.

One source of limitation on the frequency of intercourse is the taboos, or at least conventions, discouraging intercourse at particular times. Taboos during menstruation and pregnancy, which seem to have been neither extensive nor powerful, of course would not have any influence on reproduction. While there is evidence that a post-partum taboo on intercourse existed in some areas (e.g. Berndt and Berndt, 1964 : 127), it is more commonly observed that a married couple could resume sexual relations after only a few days or weeks (Warner, 1937 : 78; Meggitt, 1962 : 278; Goodale, 1971 : 27). It seems likely that even when there is a belief that post-parturient mothers should refrain from intercourse, there is little force in this rule (Roheim, 1933 : 252; Kaberry, 1939 : 154). Where a second wife is available, though, the constraint would be easy to observe. Now it may be argued that while older co-wives in particular receive less attention from their husbands, they may have lovers. The major consideration here is privacy, and this is a factor that seems to be in need of reassessment.

Privacy for sexual intercourse is of importance in all human societies. In a small hunter-gatherer group, where life is lived in public, where solitude is avoided and where everyone is aware of the activities of others, privacy is difficult to achieve. Women can use this fact to avoid intercourse. But it seems also that lack of privacy might mean a less than optimal level of sexual activity for optimal fertility, at least for some women and perhaps for all. Married couples, especially men with new young wives, frequently go out for a few days hunting together. This does seem to indicate that they have insufficient privacy normally. A woman who has one or two children may have difficulty even in finding opportunity to achieve privacy with her husband.

It seems probable that monogamously married women would not have reduced chances of conception due to low frequency of intercourse. Polygamously married women, and especially older co-wives and widows, may well have suffered, or perhaps enjoyed such a reduction in the probability of conception. Changed conditions on missions, government reserves and cattle-stations have added to the opportunity for privacy. This is obviously so in places where houses are available. Also with the reduced level of hunting and gathering, and with larger groups collected in one place, there is more leisure and more opportunity for autonomy and thus privacy. A further factor of some importance is that the traditional severe punishments for illicit liaisons have been suppressed by European law-enforcement agents. These factors would be likely to have a major effect on the frequency and regularity of intercourse.

Male Fertility

The fact that it is older men who traditionally had regular and licit access to the most fertile women makes the fertility of older men of interest. Male fertility does gradually decrease with age to some extent, but unlike women, men seldom completely lose their fertility. It is widely recognized that Aboriginal men's ability to enforce the fidelity of their young wives is limited. However, the reduced level of fertility in these old men would have had some influence on the conception rate, since their control over their wives did severely curtail the access of these women to younger men.

Early observers viewed sub-incision,[4] which is practised over large areas of south, central and Western Australia, as the Australian Aborigines' successful solution to the Malthusian problem. Later writers became convinced that sub-incision was not intended as a contraceptive device, and indeed did not interfere with conception. While it is clearly the case that sub-incision was not intended for contraceptive purposes, it does seem that it would have had the effect of reducing the probability of conception to some extent. Sub-incision is a source of blood for rituals, as well as being the occasion for ritual. The incision is extended at each ceremony, so that there would be an increased contraceptive effect at the later stages. Older men, who monopolize women, thus would be most affected. A second factor concerning male genital operations is the increased likelihood of urethral stricture caused either by infection or by scarring. This is likely to lead to sterility in men. However, as sub-incision has never been practised over large areas of eastern Australia, nor in Arnhem Land, it cannot account for the pre-contact birth spacing in these areas.

Finally, a myth reported by Howitt (1904 : 796) tells of the inflammation of a man's penis when he continued sexual activity after being circumcised. His immodest behaviour enraged others and they killed him. It seems likely that the reference is in fact to sub-incision, either the original operation, the extension of the incision or the reopening of the wound for the supply of blood for ritual purposes. The myth implies that there is a period of abstinence after such operations, no doubt because of the painfulness of intercourse at such times. Any such abstinence at regular intervals should be noted as causing some reduction in the conception rate.

FACTORS AFFECTING GESTATION

Finally, to complete this examination of factors affecting Australian Aboriginal fertility, we must examine the probability that conception will not result in a birth: that is, the probability of spontaneous abortion. It has been noted that a possible consequence of abortion is sterility caused by oviduct blockage. The rate of spontaneous abortion is a good deal higher in all populations than is generally known. According to one study in the United States, one-third of all fertilized ova are shed before the first missed period; another estimate from the United Kingdom shows that 48 per cent of zygotes suffer early or late foetal loss (Nurge, 1975 : 26; James, 1975 : 1). Environmental conditions influence this rate, especially during the 8–19 week gestation period (Cutright, 1975 : 424). The rate of spontaneous foetal loss changes over time in response to changing environmental conditions. It seems probable that the major environmental conditions that would increase the rate of foetal wastage among Australian Aborigines are the physical demands of food collection in harsh climatic conditions and a somewhat irregular diet, including a high percentage of roughage. Though there is no experimental support for this assertion, it seems intuitively probable that such conditions would increase considerably the rate of foetal wastage.

DISCUSSION

This paper has attempted to demonstrate that birth rates among Australian Aborigines were traditionally low because of environmental and social conditions of various kinds. The importance of this review in the light of current problems will be discussed briefly.

Aborigines consider few and well spaced children normal, and it is against this underlying and relatively constant background that conscious attempts at reproductive control must be seen. Thus, for instance, pregnancies in Aboriginal girls before twenty years are often seen as abnormal, improper and dangerous, as are pregnancies in older women, and most importantly, pregnancies occurring too soon after the birth of an infant.

Reproductive desires in any society are the primary factor determining the use of introduced contraceptive services. That is, people will use new techniques only to achieve previously desired aims. While little research has been done into the reproductive aims of Aborigines, there are indications that the women at least are eager to control their birth-rate.[5] The Goinjimbi women are concerned and upset when young girls become pregnant, for they are seen to be not strong enough to bear and rear a child. Even more anxiety is expressed when a woman who is still suckling becomes pregnant. Both the mother and the older baby are seen to be under severe stress. In this situation, it is felt that one of the children will inevitably suffer, since a mother cannot produce sufficient milk for both. The foetus is seen as a threat to the health of mother and infant, and the suckling infant is considered to have prior claim on the mother's milk. A mother feels that she is denying the infant its valid rights when attempting to wean it for the sake of the coming baby, and thus suffers guilt and anxiety.

Aboriginal attitudes towards the nurturance of infants and spacing of births differ markedly from conventional attitudes in white society. Many doctors and nurses consider the first child quite able to survive without the mother's milk, and normally do not advise the mother about how this can be achieved. A better understanding of the intense protectiveness and attachment towards suckling infants up to three and four years of age should equip health personnel to deal with problems resulting from closely spaced births. This is a recent situation, which is poorly understood by both Aborigines and whites alike. Aboriginal cultural practices have not yet adapted to deal with the changed situation. It is to be hoped that the information in this paper may aid in the achievement of a better adjustment and of a more effective and responsible health service for Aboriginal women.

ACKNOWLEDGEMENTS

This study is based on literature research and on field observations made at Goinjimbi in southern Arnhem Land in 1975, 1976 and 1979. The author is grateful to the members of that community for their support and friendship, and to Annette Hamilton, Les Hiatt, John Murray (gynaecologist) and Janice Reid for useful comments and criticisms. The data and issues discussed in this paper are presented in greater detail in Cowlishaw, 1979.

NOTES

1 The argument is not, of course, that the diet is "better", but that the specific effect of increased fertility might be associated with an increased calorific intake and less roughage.

2 It may be suggested that the low body fat indicating lack of energy reserves discussed above may increase the anovulatory effect of lactation. However, malnourished women, eating little protein, produce breast milk of relatively normal protein content for long periods (Bailey, 1965 : 47). It seems rather that the effect is the other way around. Lack of energy causes anovulation and this effect may be increased during lactation, as Frisch (1978) states.

3 Women do this not as a consequence of any biologically given difference in sexual receptivity, but as a direct result of the socialization of women's sexuality. See Cowlishaw, 1979.

4 Ceremonial incision to open underside of penis to urethra along its length.

5 See especially Reid and Gurruwiwi (1979), who found that Aboriginal women often want and would accept contraception, but are effectively unable to obtain such help because of the culturally unacceptable, often humiliating way in which such services are offered.

REFERENCES

Abbie, A. A., 1960. "Physical Changes in Australian Aborigines Consequent Upon European Contact", *Oceania* 31, no. 2 : 140–44.

Ackerman, K., 1975. "Altered Food Taboos", *Oceania* 46, no. 2 : 122–25.

Bailey, K. V., 1965. "Quantity and Composition of Breast Milk in some New Guinean Populations", *Journal of Tropical Pediatrics* 11, no. 2 : 35–48.

Barwick, D. E., 1971. "Changes in Aboriginal Population of Victoria,

1863–1966", in *Aboriginal Man and Environment in Australia*, ed. D. J. Mulvaney and J. Golson (Canberra : Australian National University Press), pp. 288–315.

Becroft, Thelma C., 1967. "Child-rearing Practices in the Highlands of New Guinea: A Longitudinal Study of Breast Feeding", *Medical Journal of Australia* 2, no. 13 : 598–601.

Berndt, R. M., and Berndt, C. H., 1943. "Fieldwork in Western South Australia", *Oceania* 13, no. 3 : 243–80.

——— and ———, 1964. *The World of the First Australians* (Sydney : Ure Smith).

Billington, B. P., 1960. "The Health and Nutritional Status of the Aborigines", in Mountford (1960), pp. 27–55.

Cowlishaw, G. K., 1978. "Infanticide in Aboriginal Australia", *Oceania* 48, no. 4 : 262–83.

———, 1979. "Women's Realm: A Study of Socialization, Sexuality and Reproduction among Australian Aborigines" (Ph.D. thesis, University of Sydney).

Cutright, P., 1975. "Spontaneous Fetal Loss: A Note on Rates and Some Implications", *Journal of Biosocial Science* 7 : 421–33.

Delvoye, P., Delogne-Desnoeck, J., and Robyn, C., 1976. "Serum Pro-lactin in Long-lasting Lactation Amenorrhoea", *Lancet* 2 : 288–89.

Fomon, S. J., 1967. *Infant Nutrition* (Philadelphia : Saunders).

Frisch, Rose E., 1978. "Population, Food Intake and Fertility", *Science* 199 : 22–30.

——— and McArthur, Janet W., 1974. "Menstrual Cycles: Fatness as a Determinant of Minimum Weight for Height Necessary for their Maintenance or Onset", *Science* 185 : 949–51.

Goodale, J. C., 1971. *Tiwi Wives* (Seattle : University of Washington Press).

Healy, D. L., and Burger, H. G., 1977. "Review: Human Prolactin — Recent Advances in Physiology and Therapy", *A.N.Z. Journal of Obstetrics and Gynaecology* 17, no. 2 : 61–78.

Hernandez, T., 1941. "Children Among the Drysdale River Tribes", *Oceania* 12, no. 2 : 122–33.

Hiatt, L. R., 1978. "Genealogies of Anbarra Population", unpublished ms. (Canberra : Australian Institute of Aboriginal Studies).

Himes, Norman E., 1936. *Medical History of Contraception* (Baltimore : Williams & Wilkins).

Howell, N., 1976. "The Population of the Dobe Area !Kung", in Lee and De Vore (1976), pp. 136–51.

Howitt, A. W., 1904. *Native Tribes of South-East Australia* (London : Macmillan).

James, W. H., 1975. "The Fitness of the Human Zygote", *Journal of Biosocial Science* 7 : 1–4.

Jones, F. L., 1963. *A Demographic Survey of the Aboriginal Population of the Northern Territory with Special Reference to Bathurst Island Mission* (Canberra : Australian Institute of Aboriginal Studies).

Kaberry, P., 1939. *Aboriginal Woman: Sacred and Profane* (London : Routledge & Sons).

Krzywicki, L. 1934. *Primitive Society and Its Vital Statistics* (London: Macmillan).
Lee, R. B., and De Vore, I. (eds), 1968. *Man the Hunter (Chicago: Aldine).*
—— and —— (eds), 1976. *Kalahari Hunter-Gatherers* (Cambridge, Mass.: Harvard University Press).
Llewellyn-Jones, D., 1972. *Everywoman* (London: Faber & Faber).
McArthur, M., 1960. "Food Consumption and Dietary Levels of Groups of Aborigines Living on Naturally Occurring Foods", in Mountford (1960), pp. 90–135.
McCarthy, F. D., and McArthur, M., 1960. "The Food Quest and the Time Factor in Aboriginal Economic Life", in Mountford (1960), pp. 145–94.
Meehan, B., 1975. "Shell Bed to Shell Midden" (Ph.D. thesis. Department of Prehistory and Anthropology, Australian National University, Canberra).
Meggitt, M. J., 1962. *Desert People* (Sydney: Angus & Robertson).
Mountford, C. G. (ed.), 1960. *Records of the American–Australian Scientific Expedition to Arnhem Land*, vol. 2, *Anthropology and Nutrition* (Melbourne: Melbourne University Press).
Nag, Moni, 1962. *Factors Affecting Human Fertility in Non-industrial Societies: A Cross-cultural Study*, Yale University Publications in Anthropology, no. 66 (New Haven: Yale University Press).
——, 1972. "Sex, Culture and Human Fertility: India and the United States", Current Anthropology 13, no. 2: 231–37.
Nurge, E., 1975. "Spontaneous and Induced Abortion in Human and Non-human Primates", in *Being Female: Reproduction, Power and Change*, ed. D. Raphael (The Hague: Mouton), pp. 25–35.
Peterson, J. N., 1972. "The Structure of Two Australian Aboriginal Ecosystems" (Ph.D. thesis, University of Sydney).
Reid, J. C., and Gurruwiwi, M., 1979. "Attitudes towards Family Planning among the Women of a Northern Aboriginal Community", *Medical Journal of Australia (Special Supplement)* 1, no. 2: 5–7.
Roheim, G., 1933. "Women and Their Life in Central Australia", *Journal of Royal Anthropological Institute of Great Britain and Ireland* 63: 207–65.
Rose, F., 1968. "Australian Marriage. Land-owning Groups and Initiations", in Lee and De Vore (1968), pp. 200–208.
Roth, W. E., 1908. "Marriage Ceremonies and Infant Life", *North Queensland Ethnography Bulletin No. 10*, in *Records of the Australian Museum* 7: 1–17.
Sharp, L., 1940. "An Australian Aboriginal Population", *Human Biology* 12: 281–507.
Spencer, W. B., and Gillen, F. J., 1968. *The Native Tribes of Central Australia* (New York: Dover; first published 1899).
Stanner, W. E. H., 1933. "The Daly River Tribes: A Report of Field Work in North Australia", *Oceania* 4: 10–29.
Tanner, J. M., 1968. "Earlier Maturation in Man", *Scientific American* 218, no. 1: 21–27.
Tonkinson, R., 1978. "Semen versus Spirit-Child in a Western Desert Culture", in *Australian Aboriginal Concepts*, ed. L. R. Hiatt (New Jersey: Humanities Press), pp. 81–92.

Warner, W. L., 1937. *A Black Civilization: A Social Study of an Australian Tribe* (New York : Harper & Bros.; rev. edn, 1958; Torchbook edn, 1964).

White, I. M., 1977. "Pitfalls to Avoid: The Australian Experience", in *Health and Disease in Tribal Societies*, Ciba Foundation Symposium 49 (Amsterdam : Elsevier, Excerpta Medica), pp. 269–301.

Yengoyan, A. A., 1972. "Biological and Demographic Components in Aboriginal Australian Socio-economic Organisation", *Oceania* 43, no. 2 : 85–95.

3
Child Health and Child Care in a Desert Community, 1970–1971

Annette Hamilton

The way in which infants and children receive their earliest impressions of the society in which they live has been largely neglected in anthropological literature. Early studies in the "culture and personality" school (exemplified by the work of Whiting & Child, 1953) were strongly influenced by an often crude understanding of Freudian theory, and attempted, by an analysis of toileting, feeding practices and similar adult-to-child training techniques, to establish the foundations on which adult personality rested in different cultural systems. The lack of notable theoretical success in this field led to a lapse of anthropological interest in the field of child-rearing as a whole, and the study of children was left largely to psychologists, especially to those concerned with establishing cross-cultural norms in child development (see, for example, Berry & Dasen, 1974).

Child-rearing among Australian Aborigines was similarly neglected. Apart from a few short papers (e.g. Hernandez, 1941; Goodale, 1960) and passing references in general works, there was in 1967 no single study devoted to rearing and education of Aboriginal children, either under pre- or post-colonial conditions. During fieldwork carried out at the Maningrida settlement, north-central Arnhem Land, in 1967–68, the author came to focus on the question of child-rearing as the central aspect of study (see Hamilton, 1981). Since that time, little new material has been published (although there is a useful discussion in Berndt and Berndt, 1972) and a broadly based understanding of Aboriginal methods of child care on a continent-wide basis, under a variety of conditions, is still lacking and is an area requiring urgent research.

The necessity of such work is not merely academic or theoretical, however. In the last decade, the state of Aboriginal infant and child health has become a significant social issue, with reports from health care professionals consistently indicating a high infant mortality rate and a high level of morbidity among Aboriginal infants and children, especially those in the remote regions of the country where links with the Aboriginal past are strongest. The child-rearing studies so far carried out indicate that Aboriginal methods of child-rearing stress the autonomy of the child in all its dealings with the social and physical environment. Adults do not "train" children, but expect them to unfold at their own pace and in their own way, with minimal interference from the adult world. Children are treated leniently and are seldom physically punished; whenever possible, they are given what they want, and are indulged by everyone in their social world. Dependency on the biological parents is diffused by links of care and responsibility towards others, articulated through the kinship system. Usually children are treated with respect and loving care.

People working among Aborigines may not see this aspect, however. Much more obvious is the fact that the children are dirty, their noses and ears frequently discharge pus, they are often thin and often ill. The apparent disjunction between Aboriginal attitudes of care and affection towards their children, and the poor state of health of those children, will form a primary focus of this paper. It is not meaningful to link practices of child care with outcome in child health without considering the environmental setting within which the child lives — or in a word, the child's ecology.

The information in this paper was obtained while carrying out fieldwork for fifteen months in 1970–71 among Janggundjara and Bidjandjara-speaking people living in a small community in the north-west of South Australia. The community was situated on a cattle-station, Everard Park, which was in private hands at the time. The station employed casual Aboriginal labour when required, but otherwise interfered little with and contributed little to the lives of the Aboriginal people, whose traditional home it had been. Everard Park subsequently was purchased by the Commonwealth government as part of Aboriginal lands, and its name changed to Mimili. In this paper, the area will be referred to as Everard Park, since that is how it was known during the author's time there and the information relates to that period only. It was a small and homogeneous community, probably similar in structure and organization to many of those currently referred to as "outstations", and the child care and child health in this community would be reasonably typical of the Western Desert regions.[1]

THE PHYSICAL ENVIRONMENT

The north-western corner of South Australia lies in the most arid region of the continent, in the belt where average rainfall is low (below 127 mm) and not reliably seasonal. It is characterized by extremes of heat and cold, summer temperatures being in excess of 43°C for days at a time, while below freezing temperatures are common on winter nights. When rain falls, it does so in drenching downpours, with little warning. Flies are myriad, and in summer cannot be controlled: eyes, nose, ears and mouth, as well as all foodstuffs, are constantly covered with them. Water still may be obtained from traditional sources, especially the large rockholes that act as reservoirs in the granite ranges and that, in the past, provided a refuge for both animals and people in the ranges area; since pastoral settlement, it has been provided also from bores that tap the underground water-table and may be of poor quality. Today, as in the past, periods of drought alternate with periods of relative plenty. At Everard Park itself, rainfall records show that, from 1950 to 1971, there was a constant fluctuation of annual rainfall.

There were periods of absolute drought: thirty-six such occasions occurred in the said period, lasting a minimum of two months up to a maximum of eight months. Drought periods mean not only the absence of fresh drinking water but also that there is little fresh vegetable food available. There is, in addition, a total reduction in the available meat supply, due to the reproductive characteristics of the desert marsupials; during drought the red kangaroo, for example, ceases to breed and pouch young die.

Although today Aborigines are no longer dependent on indigenous food and water supplies, the climatic fluctuations remain significant in determining the quality of the living environment, the availability of fresh water and the possibility of supplementing the diet with non-purchased foodstuffs, especially meat.

Of greater significance, however, is the physical living environment in which people must cook, eat, find shelter from environmental extremes, rest and care for the young, the old and the sick. In common with many "outback" Aboriginal people, the living standards in this area were very poor, although the people of the Everard camp were better off than many of their neighbours. Traditionally, shelters were used only when people expected to be camped in one place for a relatively long period of time. Shades were erected against the summer heat, and low, domed shelters of wood, with spinifex and logs, provided more substantial shelters during rainy periods. A small inside fire provided light and warmth, and food was cooked outside on fires within a windbreak, also constructed of branches and spinifex. The amount of material and labour invested in these shelters was very small; they could be shifted, rebuilt, modified and abandoned altogether with minimal disruption to other activities. A high "table" made of logs or the branch of a tree served to keep foodstuffs and other goods away from dogs.

The shelters that the people build themselves today are modelled on the same principles. However, since the people move less frequently, they tend to build more substantial shelters, and the longer they stay in one place, the less available is building material such as branches and logs. No housing was provided for the people at Everard who were not currently employed on the station, and so the unemployed followed traditional principles in constructing their shelters. One important modification, however, was the "camp-sheet", a piece of water-proof canvas stretched over the top of the shelter to keep out the rain.

No one had a frame bed, but some had mattresses and all had blankets, which were shaken out and aired frequently. All water used in the camp had to be carried in containers from the bore about three-quarters of a kilometre away; four-gallon plastic jerry-cans were the most popular. Most families were obliged to go to and from the bore twice a day; women went together in small parties, morning and evening, but men and older children also helped. There were no ablution blocks or toilet facilities. People washed themselves at the bore, and washed children in containers about ten centimetres deep, which served also for mixing damper and cooking meat. In outback Australia, they are known as "camp-ovens". Areas at the outskirts of the camp were used for defecation; people had a clear idea of "dirtiness" and indeed shifted their individual camps to a new site, or even shifted the whole camp, in response to the perception that the area was becoming fouled.[2]

Although theirs must be one of the most demanding physical habitats imaginable, the Aborigines had devised ingenious methods that allowed them to live with a modicum of comfort; certainly they were passionately attached to their country and showed no interest in leaving it or exchanging it for the apparent comforts of any other way of life. The physical landscape remained a matter of powerful spiritual import, and traditional religious and ritual life continued to flourish and to provide a meaningful background of explanation, belief and codes of conduct.

THE SOCIAL AND ECONOMIC SETTING

All members of the Everard camp were related to one another by a series of intersecting genealogical connections. The core of the camp consisted of the old men and the old women, who were mostly in receipt of aged pensions and whose authority in traditional matters was unquestioned. Some of these older people were married to one another, others were widows and widowers. Their siblings were found either in the same camp or at the adjacent settlements of Indulkana and Fregon, although some lived further away again. The sons and daughters of these older people, with their own spouses and children, moved from one area to another quite frequently, although as families grew there was a tendency to remain in the camp of either the husband's or the wife's parents. Younger, unmarried people travelled frequently from place to place, the young men working on nearby cattle-stations as stock-hands and casual labourers, the young women as domestic servants. There was no school at Everard, so the children remained in the camp with their parents, unless they accompanied them on a visit to one of the settlements where a school was available. There was a high level of mobility between areas, fostered by the purchase of motor vehicles and accentuated by occasional ceremonies. The degree of variability in camp numbers can be seen in Figure 1 below.

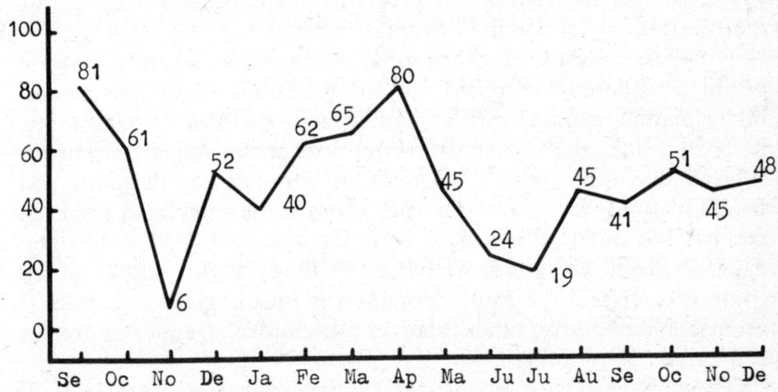

Fig. 1. Everard Park (Mimili), Total Monthly Population, Permanent Residents, September 1970-December 1971

These patterns of mobility have very serious implications for the way in which significant resources, especially money and food, are distributed, and for the way in which these resources can be used for those most in need of care. The balance of men, women and children, and young and old, in any camp determines the effectiveness with which the healthy and able-bodied can care for the young, the old and the sick. The presence of too many old and infirm people in a camp places intense pressure on young women especially, who also are most likely to be those caring for young and often sick children. The expectation of care from relatives means that no "family" can ever be considered in isolation from others, and the human labour necessary to sustain healthy human life falls much more heavily on some than on others, especially in the absence of our so readily taken for granted Western amenities and welfare facilities.

On the other hand, Aborigines generally are able to rely on a large number of relatives to provide them with goods and services, when available. Money and food obtained by one person will not necessarily be for the use of his or her immediate family: other obligations may require that goods are distributed in other directions. For example, a man may have to make payments in money to other men in connection with ritual obligations, even though this may mean that his wife and children have nothing at all and must find assistance from other relatives. The contractual obligations arising out of marriage are seen primarily as between a woman's husband and her parents, rather than between husband and wife, while women are considered primarily responsible for obtaining the food necessary for their young children.

For these reasons, the Aboriginal communities of this area cannot be considered a collection of nuclear families; attempts to correlate "family income" with any other factors would be misleading. In 1970, for example, a study carried out at the Amata settlement showed that there was no correlation between health status and family income. A total income per month was calculated for each family, "but did not include . . . money acquired 'by family right' from relatives" (Fergin & Melville, 1970 : 4). If this source of income is excluded, the figure obtained is meaningless. Not only is money obtained from other relatives but children frequently are fed and cared for by others.

The sources of cash income for the Everard people were, in 1970 and 1971, limited indeed. Income was derived largely from government-paid pensions to the old-aged and invalid, child endowment to mothers, and occasional wage-labour on the station. Most adult men were unemployed most of the year. In 1971, only four men were regularly employed and entitled to unemployment benefit, and one of these lived permanently away from the camp and contributed little cash to the community.

In 1971, considering income from all sources (a total of $22 178), the cash income per head was $14.20 per fortnight or $369.20 per head per year. (The total population was taken as fifty permanent residents and ten visitors.) By comparison with figures for mission and government settlement desert communities, the Everard group was at the upper end of the scale. Peterson (1978 : 33) provides the following figures:

Income per head per two-week period in 1970

	$
Warburton	4.55
Ernabella	8.49
Amata	11.97
Yuendumu	11.72
Docker River	14.43

In 1970–71, unemployment benefits were not widely paid to Aborigines on missions and settlements, which may account in part for the relative wealth of the cattle-station groups. On the other hand, in white Australia, the gross domestic product figure per head per fortnight was $99.39 ($2584 per annum).[3]

During the period of fieldwork, there was no permanent store in the Everard camp. People received their pension money from a vehicle that travelled from Indulkana, known as "the patrol", which usually was driven by a nursing sister, who examined the health of the people at the same time. The sister sold infant food and eggs, fruit and goods such as camp-sheets, soap and clothing. After she left, the homestead "store" appeared on the back of a truck, from which all staples such as flour, tea and sugar would be purchased. Money was received fortnightly and people would then make the bulk of their purchases, keeping enough for a smaller number of purchases the following week. There was no regular supply of fresh meat, and all significant protein sources were gained from hunting and gathering. The approximate cash value of meat supplied by hunting was calculated, on the basis of 40 cents per pound (453 g)[4] of meat, as $4009 for the year.

A number of estimates of money spent on purchased goods, and the nature of these goods, has been made over different periods of time. The following figures are based on a monitoring of purchases during two two-week periods, the first beginning 19 January, and the second 4 March 1971. The total purchases made by all community members from all sources during that period, together with the amount of money received from social services and the amount of money spent, have been recorded. (During each period approximately 420 lb (190.3 kg) of meat was procured by hunting.) From these figures, it is possible to estimate the average approximate consumption of selected items per fortnight and per day. (The total population has been taken as 53, excluding the 15 babies and children under four years, who have been used as the population for the milk and baby-food figures.)

Average Consumption of Selected Food Items

Item	Total in 4-week period	Per head per 2-week period		Per day	
	(lb)	(lb)	(kg)	(lb)	(gm)
flour	875	8.3	3.74	0.59	267.0
meat (hunted)	840	7.9	3.59	0.57	256.0
sugar	232	2.2	0.99	0.16	70.0
tea	26	0.25	0.11	0.02	8.0
jam	14	0.13	0.06	0.01	4.3
potatoes	59	0.56	0.25	0.04	18.0
milk	34	1.1	0.51	0.08	36.7
eggs	552	5.21		0.37	
oranges	160	1.51		0.11	
baby-food	242 tins	8.06 tins		0.58 tins	

These admittedly approximate figures none the less give some idea of the dietary habits of the people. The daily consumption of flour is relatively low compared to that at some other communities. Peterson (1977) reports that at Warburton in 1970, people were consuming white flour at the rate of 604 g per head per day, and at Amata, it was 408 g per head (cf. 267 g at Everard Park). Because additional food brought in by visitors has not been included here, the estimates will be somewhat low. However, it seems likely that the higher the *per capita* income, and the greater the availability of meat (either from hunting or by purchase), the less will be the reliance on white flour as a dietary staple.

Foods such as jam, eggs, oranges and potatoes were all consumed within a day or two of their purchase, and only flour, sugar and tea would be kept over from one purchase to the next. People also procured a variable quantity of wild vegetable foods, as well as small protein sources such as goanna eggs, witchetty-grubs, and so on. The figures for baby-food and milk are approximate also, since they include in the averaging small babies, who would receive little supplementary feeding, and children up to the age of four, who would also receive other food. It will be apparent that children who are reliant on purchased food alone will be extremely undernourished.

The whole adjustment of the Everard community rested on the continuation of hunting and gathering. For this reason, relatively little of the cash income was spent on food, or indeed was spent at all. In fact, during the first two-week period monitored, only 46 per cent of the available income was spent at all ($217.95 of $474) and in the second period, 68 per cent was spent ($272.05 of $400). The remaining money was disbursed in two ways. A proportion was sent by parents to their adult children living at other settlements, especially at Indulkana. About 18 per cent was accounted for in this way. The balance was saved as cash, in order to contribute to the cost of motor vehicles, for which this community saved constantly. Between September 1970 and December 1971, one truck costing $1500 was purchased as the collective property of the community, and three smaller cars were purchased. This pattern of relatively small expenditure on food also was found by Anderson (1976) at Amata in 1975, where between 55 and 59 per cent of money was spent on food.

This account provides the background against which the nature of child-care and child health in this remote desert community must be understood. The physical and social environment, and the economic system, together provide the "material" structure within which the Aboriginal child's life is lived. The other side of the picture is provided by the attitudes, values and beliefs of the community about adults and children, illness and health. These aspects are expressed in concrete practices, which can be observed in people's daily lives as the totality of methods of care.

THE CHILDREN

Children are a central part of life in the desert communities; they are always visible and audible, and lead a free and indulged existence, which contrasts with the careful deportment and modest demeanour of the adults. People refer to them collectively as *djidji djurda* (the children), including all those from toddlers up to the age when boys are segregated to await their initiation and girls are incorporated into the lives of adult women, even if not yet married. The focus of this paper, however, is the younger children, particularly those under five years of age. We begin with a description of their health, giving case examples to illustrate the commonalities — and differences — in their social and medical circumstances.

Child Health

As mentioned, the level of mobility between areas is high, and many children spend equal periods of time at more than one place. However, there was a small group of stable residents at Everard Park whose children usually were to be found in the Everard camp. There were sixteen of these children aged under five and their "vital statistics" are summarized below, by age.

No.	Sex	Age in Months (July 1971)	Height (cm)	Weight (kg)	Haemoglobin[a] (August 1971)
1	male	1	n.a.	3.01	n.a.
2	male	3	n.a.	4.06	10.5
3	male	10	73	9.00	8.5
4	male	14	84	10.15	n.a.
5	female	16	72	9.32	6.5
6	female	17	80	9.10	n.a.
7	female	18	82	9.96	6.0
8	male	28	83	10.82	11.0
9	female	29	n.a.	11.36	11.0
10	female	30	87	12.00	7.0
11	female	32	85	10.30	8.5
12	female	36	91	13.10	11.0
13	male	36	90	15.00	12.0
14	male	38	100	13.27	9.0
15	male	54	99	13.30	11.0
16	male	58	99	14.30	6.5

(a) Data derived from a field assay of haemoglobin levels carried out by the South Australian Department of Health. Figures represent grams per 100 ml.

In Figure 2 below, the weights of these children are charted against the standard weight chart used by the Department of Health to assess the progress of Aboriginal (and other) children. This gives at a glance the usual index used to assess how well a child is "thriving". Children in this community followed the usual pattern of Aboriginal child growth, as is now well established from studies such as those by Maxwell and Elliott (1969), Jose and Welch (1970) and Kirke (1969, 1971). Aboriginal infants generally are born at a lower birth weight than white infants (cf. Parsons, 1965; Kettle, 1966), but grow rapidly until the age of four or five months, often catching up with or passing the weight of white infants. After this period, the rate of weight gain slows or stops altogether, as does the height gain to a lesser extent. Children remain well below "standards" until the age of six or so, and then the growth curve begins to tend upwards again. This pattern is now well established for Aboriginal children in different environments in many parts of the continent, although the extent of growth retardation among the south-central Australian people is greater than that in the northern part of the Northern Territory or in northern Queensland (cf. Moodie, 1973 : 182). It is now widely accepted that many of these children are malnourished and manifest the symptoms of protein–calorie malnutrition. Maxwell and Elliott, 1969. The same authors note that Aboriginal children fostered in white homes approximated white norms in their growth patterns, so there is nothing to suggest that the Aboriginal infants' growth patterns are part of a genetic heritage). Malnutrition occurs in conjunction with repeated episodes of infection: gastro-enteritis, otitis media and acute respiratory tract infections are the most common.

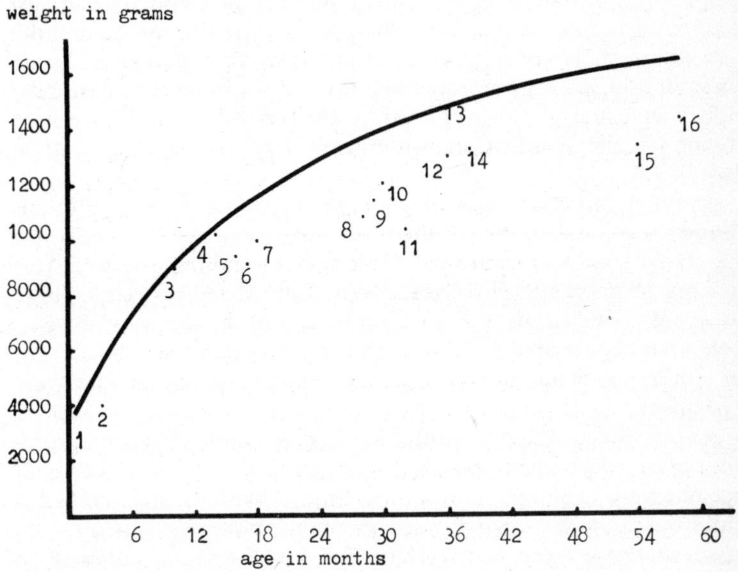

Fig. 2. Everard Park Children : Weights by Age

Source: After Commonwealth of Australia, Department of Health; approximation, normal weight curve, 60 months.

The haemoglobin levels reported here show a similar pattern to those found among Aboriginal children elsewhere. A minimum "safe" level of 11 g per 100 ml of blood has been suggested as appropriate for Aboriginal children up to the age of four years (cf. Moodie, 1973 : 192). Researchers have found that Aboriginal children have levels up to 2 g below those regarded as standard for white children at all ages from six months to twelve years. Moodie (1973:194) concludes that anaemia in Aboriginal children is "from ten to twenty times as common as in the white population, and is more often severe".

Many of the Aboriginal children of Everard Park manifested then a number of classic symptoms of chronic ill-health. It is of some interest to consider a few of their stories in some detail, before turning to a consideration of the practices of child care in this community.

We will start with the children (3, 4 and 13) whose weights appeared to be closest to the norm.

Child 3: Although his weight was at the norm, this child was below the norm in height and his haemoglobin level was low. His weight was as it was because he had been hospitalized due to repeated illnesses since he was three months old, and he had just returned from the most recent episode. He was an unwanted child, and although his unmarried teenage mother refused to give him up for adoption, he was not well cared for and could be considered the only "neglected" child in the camp. He certainly would have died if not for the concern and intervention of the medical staff at Indulkana.

Child 4, however, was a healthy and much loved child; his mother was the daughter of the most important ritual custodian in the camp and was active in women's ceremonials herself. Her parents both received pensions, as did her husband's parents. There were only three children in the family, and both parents were competent and concerned with their children's welfare, making a point of purchasing foods such as eggs and oranges whenever they were available.

Child 13 was an only child. His mother had been married previously to a European, who had deserted her, and the children of the marriage had been placed in welfare homes in Adelaide.[5] This child was from her second marriage to an Aboriginal man and was a substitute for those she had lost. She was also better educated in nutrition than most of the other women in the camp. However, she tended to overfeed the child, who was visibly fat and provided a heavy burden to the mother and other relatives when he needed to be carried.

At the other extreme were children 5, 6, 11, 15 and 16. Child 6 was much loved, but her parents' concern could not seem to avert the frequent bouts of respiratory infections and otitis media that she experienced. She had never been so ill as to require hospitalization, but had received repeated courses of antibiotics and appeared to be going into a weight decline. Child 11 barely survived 1971. She had been born close to a previous sibling (twenty-two months was the interval between them); the sibling was Child 15, and the mother obviously was unable to care for them both adequately. Others said it was because they were "too close"; the mother herself blamed her husband for the health of the children, saying that he spent too much time on ritual matters and too little money on food. Usually he was unemployed and often absent from the camp; his position as the son of an important ritual leader necessitated his frequent travels. The little girl became seriously ill with diarrhoea during August 1971, when the family was attending ceremonies at Fregon. Not knowing the medical staff there personally, the mother would not take the child for attention and instead demanded that her husband take them back to Everard. But the husband could not do this, due to his involvement in the ceremonies, and so he refused. The mother had been told by nursing sisters that a child with diarrhoea should not be fed, so she gave the child nothing but sugared water and unfortunately continued this treatment for four days, while the child's condition deteriorated. At last the father became alarmed, and they travelled to Indulkana with the child in a prostrate condition. She was hospitalized in Alice Springs after emergency evacuation and subsequently recovered, but remained tiny and fragile. Her older brother had had a similar medical history in his first two years of life, but had survived and now appeared to be active and wiry, although suffering from chronic nasal and ear discharge.

Child 16 and Child 5 were brother and sister. Although both children were below growth standards, they appeared healthy and active. Both children's haemoglobin levels were alarmingly low, as were those of their other two siblings, all of whom were tested with levels of between 6 and 7 g. Their mother's level was adequate, and the father's was high at 14.5. This family previously had lived on a mission station where the clinic took some responsibility for the provision of milk, bottles and supplementary food for infants. It seemed at times that this mother was reluctant to spend any money on food for the children, and she became angry and aggressive when white people refused to give her milk and porridge when she requested it.

The cases discussed here represent a considerable range of situations and events that would be typical of life in Aboriginal camps in this area, especially those away from centralized services such as schools, stores and hospitals. No simple deductions can be drawn from the children's growth records, although they certainly provide a means of immediately identifying those children who might be in need of special care. It is not justifiable, however, to deduce the relative level of care and neglect in individual cases; each child's life situation differed, as did its parents' access to material and social resources and their abilities to care for the child. Nevertheless, a constant connection with food and feeding seems to be apparent, both in the health or illness of the children, and in the parents' and others' conscious perceptions of the situation.

It is undeniable that these children, judging by normal clinical parameters, were distressingly unhealthy. Yet they seemed to be alert, active and happy, except when actually in the midst of an episode of illness; and their parents did not have any consciousness that the children were unhealthy, except when they were manifestly ill. It might be easy for an observer in this community to conclude that the children were in this state because of real parental neglect, but while we cannot dispute the poverty of their material life, their emotional and social lives were such as to make the idea of "neglect" wholly inappropriate. This was made especially apparent by the single case of real neglect discussed above; the child in question was often to be seen sitting entirely alone in the dust, howling at the top of his voice, while all around him people carried on their daily activities in complete disregard. No such behaviour would be thinkable where a "legitimate" child was concerned.

Child Care

Child care in Aboriginal groups may be, and often has been, loosely characterized as "permissive". This very imprecise term does little to explicate the methods of dealing with infants and children in these communities, and even less to show how caring is integrated into a total behavioural pattern that is expected from all adults to all children.

Firstly, a child must be accepted by the community in order to be adequately cared for. It is not simply the decision of the mother or someone else that makes a child "wanted". A group consensus must exist concerning the appropriateness of that particular child for the community. People say that a child must be *ngabardji* with its kinfolk (*walydja*), meaning there must be a mutual relevance between them. In the past, women who did not want a particular child could, and occasionally did, commit infanticide; more often, children were not born close together, and all children were wanted. None the less many died, and each child's survival into healthy adulthood was something of a miracle (as it is today also, though for rather different reasons). However, because the group as a whole took a share of the responsibility for the well-being of the children, they had to be accepted, and unacceptable children were those born to parents who were not at the time correctly married to one another (in accordance with the rules of the kinship system) and those who had been born too close to a previous sibling. Each child was breast-fed for three or four years, and the older child "with a name" was given preference.[6]

If a child meets these conditions, a number of people other than the mother and father accept specific responsibilities for the child's well-being. The grandparents are particularly important in the care of the child, and may chastise neglectful parents verbally or even strike them (behaviour that is inappropriate between members of alternate generations, that is between grandparents and grandchildren). The role of the father in child care is very noticeable among these people; fathers carry their small children about with them, feed them, talk and sing to them, entertain them with sand-drawings and stories, and even cook special foods for them, when they are available. This is in marked contrast to the relative lack of involvement of fathers in the care of small children in Arnhem Land (see Hamilton, 1981) and suggests that the division of labour in childcare between men and women may differ markedly in different Aboriginal communities.

While specified relatives have particular responsibilities towards the small child, the question of authority, that is the ability and the right to control the infant's and child's behaviour in specific ways is not so easily settled. Physical punishment is unheard of. No act by a child of five or under could conceivably provoke deliberate violence against it by its own parents. Older children might hit a child, but this is deplored, and the father especially is likely to react with anger against the older child. Here, as in Arnhem Land, the rule of thumb in dealing with children tends to be always, "give the child whatever it cries for".

There is no concept or word for "naughtiness" as such. Children who do not heed the demands or requests of others are described as *gawagawa*, which means figuratively mad, silly, thoughtless. (Literally, it is the term applied to bent things, such as boomerangs or creek-beds.) Children do not have a reputation for being *gawagawa*, although specific types of behaviour might evoke this term. Conflicts between adults and children are rare, as are conflicts between children. When one child cries for something another one has, the possessor is exhorted to pity the other, often in the terms: "*Ngaldudjara, juwa!*" – "Poor thing! Give it to him." – thus invoking the pervasive ethic of compassion for those who express a need. Compassion towards the needy is the central tenet of child-rearing philosophy, and crying is the expression of need. There is no idea that to express a wish in this way is different from the expression of a need. In fact, the one term, *muguringanji*, expresses simultaneously "to like", "to want" and "to need". Thus the concept of "spoiling" is utterly inapplicable or indeed unthinkable to Aboriginal parents.

The level of harmonious interaction between small children and others is very high. They are included in all aspects of secular life, carried about and handed around, and although they sometimes must represent a great burden to their families when the mother is caring for a number of other children as well as aged relatives, one never hears expressions of disaffection about children. When asked what the ideal number of children in a family is, the answer is invariably the number of children that that particular mother has, although women do state very clearly that it is bad to have too many, because it is too hard to feed them all properly.

Children are totally integrated into all aspects of daily community life. No special separate arrangements are made for them; they simply fit in with the needs of their parents and of the community. They may separate themselves off for a time into small groups, and then rejoin the adults, always without hindrance or any effort at controlling their behaviour, and no suggestion that they represent a difficulty or inconvenience. Adults go to extremes to avoid causing children unhappiness, and when this is unavoidable, as when an adult wishes to travel by vehicle without the children, their rage and frustration is allowed free play. Only when men and women are leaving for their sacred ceremonial grounds must the children comport themselves with subdued resignation, something that is imbued in them from the earliest age, thus marking off the realm of the ritual life from the realm of the secular in the most decisive of terms.

A general description such as the above cannot convey the multitude of behaviours between adults and small children that exist to comfort the children, to amuse them, to let them experience day by day the degree to which they are accepted and cared for within the community as a whole. How, then, can it be that these children are among the least fortunate in Australia as far as their physical health and well-being are concerned? If they are loved and cared for by their parents and others, how can they represent the segment of the

Australian population with the highest mortality and possibly the highest morbidity rates?

The answer to this is not a simple one. It is clear that the physical environment within which these children live differs markedly from that of almost all other Australians. One need merely mention the lack of running water, of any kind of adequate washing facilities, of any mean of getting rid of garbage, the inability to store food, the lack of housing, of warm clothes and bedding, and the presence of flies, dogs and dirt, to have partly answered it. There is also the possible susceptibility of Aboriginal people to particular forms of illness, against which they may have little resistance. Specific dietetic deficiencies and inherent physical intolerances also have been suggested. Such explanations cannot be used as excuses for Aboriginal ill-health, but some such factors, such as lactose intolerance (see Moodie, 1973 : 183) or Vitamin C deficiency (see Kalokerinos, 1974) none the less may be of great significance in the perpetuation of the observed patterns.

However, there is little doubt that the health of Aboriginal children today is a direct outcome of the colonization of Aboriginal lands by white settlers, and the whole train of historical events that has ensued. While there was probably a fairly high infant mortality rate among infants in Aboriginal societies before white invasion, it would seem, from the accounts of early settlers, from early photographs (see e.g. Basedow, 1904, 1914; White, 1915) and from the recollection of older people today, that the babies who survived early infancy became healthy children and adults (barring accidents and prolonged drought, which always affected the young and the old most severely). The impact of the present situation and the existence of European medical services has meant that more children today survive, but only at the cost of continued ill-health.

One area of consistent agreement between Aborigines and Europeans alike, however, appears to be the importance of food. Whites refer to the problem as one of "protein–calorie malnutrition" and Aborigines say "the kid's crying for tucker", but basically both express the same perceptions. It is necessary then to consider feeding practices in particular as an aspect of child care that seems to be central to the problems of Aboriginal child health.

Feeding Practices

Traditional practices of infant feeding probably resulted in a relatively undernourished and somewhat growth-retarded child (at least by the standards used to measure the growth and development of European children). The Aboriginal baby's main source of nourishment was its mother's milk, and babies were not given any supplementary feeding before seven months or even later.

Mothers gave their children supplementary foods not as a nutritional measure but as an educational one. The main staple of the small child appears to have been witchetty-grubs, goannas and grass-seed dampers, usually consisting of small slivers of the white flesh and small pieces of damper to suck. Red meat was not given to children until they could walk and talk, and even then was considered too "strong" in large quantities. The main principle governing infant feeding was always that the child be allowed to decide what and when to eat. If food was available, the infant and toddler could obtain it only by crying, reaching or in other ways indicating what he or she wanted.

In camp conditions today, it will be obvious that only when the people, particularly the women, are undertaking traditional gathering pursuits will the children be receiving the types of food that would meet these criteria. Hunting by rifle has supplanted men's other hunting activities to such an extent that large quantities of red meat have replaced the greater variety of foods that men might have procured when hunting was more difficult and the gathering of small protein sources such as lizards and goannas was more rewarding. Reliance on the store and on cash purchases permits some dietary supplementation with foods suitable for children, but an inspection of the sample buying records shows that the actual quantities of foods suitable for small children were limited during the period of study. In fact, rolled oats, weet-bix with milk, baby porridge, damper and a few tins of baby-food were all that children received from their parents' purchases, together with eggs and oranges on infrequent occasions, and soft drink too frequently. It must be noted here that the range and variety of foods available in stores differ considerably from place to place and from time to time. Aborigines will buy a greater variety of fresh foods if given the opportunity, but often the only available food is of the processed type, and also the interaction between storekeepers and Aborigines is not always easy (cf. Middleton & Francis, 1976).

People think of meals in terms similar to those of Europeans, as breakfast, dinner and tea, but the staple of these meals is always damper and black tea with sugar, while other foods are consumed more or less immediately, which is not surprising considering the lack of adequate storage facilities. Good health is associated with food, but only in the sense that hunger is seen as a precursor of social disruption; there is no idea of nutritional value, although there is definitely a sense in which a balance between vegetable (*mai*) and animal (*guga*) foods is preferred (cf. Middleton & Francis,

1976 : 82). Beyond this, eating is seen as something that is pleasant and satisfies hunger, rather than as an activity having a direct link with health. Health is the outcome of good feelings, which are signalled by harmonious social relationships, the absence of fear or insecurity (for example, fear of a revenge expedition or fear of the local police); and health can only be maintained by a balance between the correct social relationships and correct observation of the required ritual behaviours.

Children from an early age are expected to take food as they want it whenever it is available, and if they want to eat damper while the parents eat other foods, then that is their own decision. Since children are most often fed because they are crying, it often happens that they take damper and tea before other food that may be being cooked is ready, and then have no appetite for it. No one ever "feeds" a child. Food is made available and children eat, or not, as they choose.

Some mothers in the Everard community used artificial feeding apparatus when they lost their breast-milk. Some of them were very careful and diligent about washing bottles and providing a correct mixture, as the nursing sister had shown them; others would find it too difficult to manage and sometimes a single large bottle of milk would be made up in the morning and drunk from all day, in spite of the bottle being left in the sun in the open. Sometimes even quite small babies would be fed on tea from a bottle, or soft drink when it was available. Clearly the introduction of bottle-feeding represents one of the most severe hazards to infant health imaginable, except in those cases where the mothers seem to have accepted the medical staff's insistence on cleanliness. Even so, it is almost impossible for bottles and teats to be sterilized in camp conditions, and the spread of gastro-intestinal illness therefore must be fostered.

Feeding practices in this community then were limited by the available material resources on the one hand and affected by beliefs about the appropriate ways of handling children on the other. Their attitudes towards the autonomy of the child precluded Aboriginal mothers from the kind of bullying directiveness with which many European mothers approach the feeding of their children, while the kind of foods available on a daily basis made it unlikely that the child's own free choice could ever provide him or her with a balanced diet. Beliefs about illness and its treatment also are disconsonant with those of European medicine, as already described for this community elsewhere (see Hamilton, 1971) and as will be apparent from a number of other contributions in this volume (especially those by Bell, Berndt and Tonkinson).

CONCLUSION

Aboriginal child health must be seen as the outcome of both material and cultural factors. It is meaningless to ask which is dominant, since the two interact in specific ways, and an increase in one area (e.g. cash income) will not mean automatically that more is spent on children's welfare. Certainly it is a very complex situation. On the other hand, the basic perception of Aboriginal parents and white professionals alike is that children often do not have enough to eat. Given the limited cash income of these communities, the often limited store facilities, and the limited ability of Aborigines who are neither literate nor numerate to deal with what money they do have in a "maximizing" fashion, the fact that children may have little to eat for days on end is hardly surprising.

Given their objective life-setting, Aboriginal parents care for their children to the best of their abilities; the determinants of the ill-health of Aboriginal infants and children are multiple and interact with one another at many levels. This is no doubt why the well-meaning intervention of European medical services, on its own, has had little notable effect on the situation. A number of innovative programmes, such as the Pitjantjatjara Homelands Medical Service at nearby Pipalyatjara (Mt Davies), have been introduced in recent years, aimed at a total community approach towards Aboriginal health. The effects of such programmes may not be seen for some time. If additional barriers to effective use of resources or a massive influx of Europeans to the area should occur in the interim, their effectiveness might be disguised by the overall deterioration of the situation. The community of Everard Park, now Mimili, and others like it, may be transformed beyond recognition a decade hence. The direction of that transformation is as difficult to anticipate as the tolerated efflorescence of the homelands movement would have been two decades ago. But there is no doubt that an improvement in the health of the children is a *sine qua non* for any adequate future. The means by which an improvement can be brought about must include an expansion of the material resource base on which Aboriginal communities increasingly are relying, as well as a continuous consideration of what the Aboriginal people themselves want that future to become.

NOTES

[1] Some of the information recorded here was originally included in a widely circulated though unpublished paper, "Socio-cultural Factors in Health among the

Pitjantjatjara". This report was written while still in the field, at the urging of the South Australian Department of Health. The Department took a strong interest in this aspect of my research and assisted generously in a number of ways, especially with the provision of a caravan (or as it turned out, two). The research project as a whole was funded by the Australian Institute of Aboriginal Studies, to whom I am most grateful.

[2] For a detailed discussion of space and shelter in Centralian camps, see O'Connell, 1977.

[3] Australian Bureau of Census and Statistics, 1974. (For a recent and detailed account of Aboriginal economic status, see Altman & Nieuwenhuysen, 1979.) It is difficult to know which figure to use as a meaningful comparison. I have followed Peterson (1977) in using g.d.p., but other indices could be more appropriate, such as average weekly earnings, or basic-wage rate (D. Penny, pers. comm.).

[4] At the time of recording these data, metric measures were not in use in Australia. Where necessary, I have converted figures to metric, but in these purchasing records it does not seem a very worthwhile exercise, since their main purpose is indicative.

[5] It was a common practice in remote areas of Australia to take half-caste children from their parents whenever any reasonable case presented itself, in the belief that these children are better candidates for "assimilation" than full-Aboriginals. Although such a policy is not now tolerated the memory of the times when police rounded up half-caste children and sent them away, never to be seen by their parents again, is still a powerful one for many Aboriginal Women.

[6] Possibly because of the likelihood of infant deaths, children were not named until they reached the age of two or three. Prior to that they were all called *idi* (baby), and if they died, the mourning ceremonies for them would be brief and simple. After naming, they became full community members. The death of a child "with a name" would be deeply mourned.

REFERENCES

Altman, J. C., and Nieuwenhuysen, J., 1979. *The Economic Status of Australian Aborigines* (Cambridge : Cambridge University Press).

Anderson, P. J., 1976. *Report on Research into Aboriginal Income Distribution and Expenditure Patterns at Yuendumu, N.T.* Typescript. (Canberra : Australian Institute of Aboriginal Studies).

Australian Bureau of Statistics, 1974. *Australia at a Glance* (Canberra : Australian Government Publishing Service).

Basedow, H., 1904. "Anthropological Notes Made on the South Australian Government North-west Prospecting Expedition, 1903", *Transactions and Proceedings of the Royal Society of South Australia* 28 : 12–51.

——, 1914. *Journal of the Government North-west Expedition, Proceedings of the Royal Geographical Society of Australasia, South Australian Branch* (Adelaide : Government Printer).

Berndt, C. H., and Berndt, R. M., 1972. "Aborigines", in *Socialization in Australia*, ed. F. J. Hunt (Sydney : Angus & Robertson), pp. 115–40.

Berry, J. W., and Dasen, P. R., 1974. *Culture and Cognition: Readings in Cross-cultural Psychology* (London : Methuen).

Elliott, R. B., Maxwell, G. M., Kneebone, G. M., and Kirke, D. K., 1969. "Lactose Digestion and Breast Feeding: A Nutritional Survey in Australian Aboriginal Infants", *Australian Paediatrics Journal* 5, no. 2 : 109–13.

Fergin, P., and Melville, R., 1970. "A Financial Background to Health Problems in Aboriginal Children" (unpublished ms., Monash University).

Goodale, J. C., 1960. "Sketches of Tiwi Children", *Expedition, Bulletin of the University Museum of the University of Pennsylvania* 2, no. 1 : 3–13.

Hamilton, A., 1971. "Socio-cultural Factors in Health among the Pitjantjatjara" (unpublished ms., circulated by Department of Health, Adelaide).

——, 1981. *Nature and Nurture: Aboriginal Child-rearing in North-central Arnhem Land* (Canberra : Australian Institute of Aboriginal Studies).

Hernandez, T., 1941. "Children Among the Drysdale River Tribes", *Oceania* 12, no. 2 : 122–33.

Jose, D. G., and Welch, J. S., 1970. "Growth Retardation, Anaemia and Infection, with Malabsorption and Infestation of the Bowel: The Syndrome of Protein–Calorie Malnutrition in Australian Aboriginal Children", *Medical Journal of Australia* 1 : 349–56.

Kalokerinos, A., 1974. *Every Second Child* (Melbourne : Nelson).

Kettle, E. S., 1966. "Weight and Height Curves for Australian Aboriginal Infants and Children", *Medical Journal of Australia* 1 : 972–77.

Kirke, D. K., 1969. "Growth Rates of Aboriginal Children in Central Australia", *Medical Journal of Australia* 2 : 1005–9.

——, 1971. "Aboriginal Infant and Toddler Mortality and Morbidity in Central Australia, 1965–1969" (M.D. thesis, University of Adelaide).

Maxwell, G. M., and Elliott, R. B., 1969. "Nutritional State of Australian Aboriginal Children", *American Journal of Clinical Nutrition* 22, no. 6 : 716–25.

Meggitt, M. J., 1962. *Desert People* (Sydney : Angus & Robertson).

Middleton, M. R., and Francis, S. H., 1976. *Yuendumu and Its Children* (Canberra : Australian Government Publishing Service).

Moodie, P. M., 1973. *Aboriginal Health*, Aborigines in Australian Society 9 (Canberra : Australian National University Press).

O'Connell, J. F., 1977. "Room to Move: Contemporary Alyawara Settlement Patterns and Their Implications for Aboriginal Housing Policy", *Mankind* 11 : 119–31.

Parsons, P. A., 1965. "Growth in a Sample of Australian Aborigines from One to Twenty-three Months of Age", *Growth* 29 : 207–11.

Peterson, N., 1977. "Aboriginal Involvement with the Australian Economy in the Central Reserve during the Winter of 1970", in *Aborigines and Change: Australia in the '70s*, ed. R. M. Berndt (Canberra : Australian Institute of Aboriginal Studies).

——, 1978. "The Traditional Pattern of Subsistence to 1975", in *The Nutrition of Aborigines in Relation to the Ecosystem of Central Australia*, ed. B. S. Hetzel and H. J. Frith, C.S.I.R.O. Symposium, Canberra, October 1976 (Melbourne : C.S.I.R.O., 1978), pp. 25–35.

White, S., 1915. "Scientific Notes on an Expedition into the North-west

Regions of South Australia", *Transactions and Proceedings of the Royal Society of South Ausralia* 39 : 707–823.

Whiting, J. W., and Child, I. L., 1953. *Child Training and Personality: A Cross-cultural Study* (New Haven : Yale University Press).

4
Defiance or Despair? Petrol-sniffing in an Aboriginal Community

Maggie Brady and Rodney Morice

There are some drug-taking behaviours that, while not strictly "illegal", are often strongly condemned. Although health usually is cited as the main cause for concern, reactions are often judgemental, laced with conventional wisdom (often inaccurate) and plagued with unsubstantiated assumptions about "underlying causes". Petrol-sniffing is one of these behaviours. It has presented health workers, community advisors and welfare officers involved with Aboriginal communities in Australia (as well as their counterparts on North American Indian reservations) with a series of apparently insoluble, and certainly frustrating dilemmas. Not the least of these has been the ironic principle that any attempt to intervene in or focus on the activity seems to encourage it (Matza, 1969 : 80). Nevertheless, communities and their advisors have devised various strategies that attempt to deflect the young sniffers from their proclivities, with varying degrees of success. Some of these will be reviewed later.

Several volatile solvents are known to be abused, but the inhalation of petrol vapour is the form of solvent abuse most common among Aboriginal children in isolated parts of the country. As with American Indians, the use of petrol is probably a problem of "isolation and circumstance, not of race . . . it is the only inhalant that is readily available to them" (Jager, 1975 : 1). Rumour has it that American servicemen based in Darwin during World War II introduced petrol-sniffing to Australia, but the earliest published reports did not appear until the mid-1960s, in the *Medical Journal of Australia* (Gold, 1963; Black, 1967). Certainly petrol-sniffing is widespread in North America (Stryde, 1977; Kaufman, 1973), and it is not unreasonable to assume that Australian children experiment with inhalants to the same degree as their American peers, with urban children using glues or solvents rather than petrol (*Sydney Morning Herald*, 30 August 1980 : 1). Reports of such widespread use cerainly challenge the common belief that only "deviant" groups of children would do such a thing.

Despite the absence of an alarming number of deaths from petrol- or glue-sniffing, the behaviour usually is seen as a medical problem[1] and, like alcoholism, it is rarely looked at sociologically. Obviously the excessive use of inhalants does constitute a medical issue, particularly with regard to petrol, for petrol contains a variable percentage of benzene, a particularly toxic hydrocarbon, and lead. Tetra-ethyl lead (TEL), which is added to petrol to give higher octane ratings and to prevent "knocking", shows an affinity for the tissues of the central nervous system and is potentially damaging to the liver, kidneys and bone marrow (Watson, 1978). TEL poisoning is an entity "separate and distinguishable from inorganic lead poisoning. TEL is significantly more toxic than inorganic lead" (Boeckx *et al.*, 1977 : 140). Inorganic lead poisoning occasionally was found in children as a result of the chewing of objects painted with lead-containing paints, and used to be associated with water supplied through lead pipes. The detrimental and irreversible effects of organic lead accumulated through petrol inhalation are documented in numerous reports (Valpey *et al.*, 1978; Bass, 1978; Boeckx *et al.*, 1977). Physical signs of TEL poisoning may not be obvious, but can include minor weight loss, increased reflexes, tremor, slow heart-rate and/or low blood pressure (Beattie *et al.*, 1972). Some reports of patients who become very ill as a result of chronic petrol-sniffing note gross disorientation and "acting crazy", gross tremors and ataxic gait (Boeckx *et al.*, 1977 : 141; Valpey *et al.*, 1978). Death associated with petrol-sniffing seems to be most often from pneumonia (Valpey *et al.*, 1978 : 508; Boeckx *et al.*, 1977 : 142), asphyxiation or "sudden sniffing death", in which the sniffer may collapse suddenly after performing some strenuous exercise (Bass, 1970). Petrol-sniffers may be in more danger of being severely burned (Collins, 1978 : 698; Schmitt and Abston, 1972 : 1022). As with drinking, neither a single bout of sniffing, nor a series, produce in the sniffer any easily identifiable long-term impairment to his or her health (MacAndrew & Edgerton, 1970 : 171).[2] But of greater concern are recent reports of significant cognitive deficits and behavioural problems in children with raised lead levels due to atmospheric pollution (Needleman *et al.*, 1979; Garnys *et al.*, 1979). These findings suggest that deleterious effects of TEL may be much more widespread than previous literature indicates.

Aboriginal children who sniff often liken the experience to getting drunk or feeling "silly". As with drinking, generalizations are often made (by others) about the "disinhibiting" effects of petrol — that it "leads to" anti-social behaviour, for instance.[3] It has been reported that some adults will sniff petrol when alcohol is not available. As with drinking, petrol-sniffing forms a social interaction usually within a group. (One white observer described a session of sniffing by Aboriginal children as having a "picnic-like" atmosphere, with a blanket neatly laid down for them to sit on.) It is an occasion for "sharing, conviviality and seeking esteem", as Beckett (1964 : 33) suggests for drinking. The distinction between chronic and intermittent petrol-sniffing is rarely made, however, a point that is of crucial importance in communities where *all* the children may at some time experiment with sniffing. It seems to be a fluctuating pursuit, and its incidence flares up and dies out, often inexplicably, a factor that makes health workers' and communities' attempts to intervene hard to evaluate.

IDEAS ON AETIOLOGY

Suggestions about the "underlying causes" for petrol-sniffing range widely, but the tendency, whether medical or sociological, is to take the "maladjustment" view. Beckett (1964 : 36) suggests that this approach "treats Aboriginal society as a mere product of the dominant white society, denying it all autonomy." He approaches drinking and even drunkenness as means of attaining certain valued ends. "Such means may not be the best imaginable, but they may be the most practical under the circumstances" (1964 : 46). This attitude is found rarely in the commentaries on sniffing among Aboriginal children, and all too frequently the "explanations" assume that sniffing is synonymous with delinquency and that both acts of "deviance" are the result of parental neglect or "poor home environment". One writer (Sargent, 1978 : 6) claims that "delinquent tendencies in Aboriginal children precede the practice of petrol sniffing and not vice versa — such tendencies arise as a result of exactly the same cause as in our own society, i.e. a poor home environment." Such statements are suspect because no such "tendency" has yet been established in a particular socio-economic group (even in our own culture). Since the 1950s, criminologists have doubted the validity of statistics on delinquency and there is now significant research evidence that crime and delinquency are not, in fact, class-specific phenomena (Cernkovitch, 1978 : 116). As sociologist David Matza (1969 : 95) said: "most people raised in poverty are not especially deviant, and those who are remain conventional in countless ways." Nurcombe (1974 : 68) matched twenty-two Aboriginal boy sniffers with twenty-two "controls" and found no significant difference in terms of type of home and family prestige. A significance showed up only in the family clan affiliations.

Notwithstanding Nurcombe's findings the family is often suggested as a major factor in Aboriginal petrol-sniffing. Among the factors proposed are the absence of food, care and concern for children (Sargent, 1978 : 6), the lack of interest shown in children by their drinking fathers (Huey, 1978), and when the father is absent, the failure of other relatives to fulfil their traditional obligations to care for certain children (Webber, 1976 : 140). However, Webber comments that, although many sniffers in Arnhem Land settlements may have absent fathers, it is unlikely that this fact alone leads to sniffing; the death or absence of the father is nowhere near the traumatic event that it is for Europeans, since other male relatives may provide support for the child.

Often suggestions about the causes of petrol-sniffing are based on an intimate knowledge of individual communities, but sometimes the reports of welfare officers and medical personnel are imbued with a subtle (and not so subtle) belief that "they" are unable to "deal with" their kids when they misbehave or sniff petrol; or that "they" are inadequate as parents. It is certainly hard to believe that the two hundred children who sniff petrol at Shamattawa, Canada, the fifty or so at Maningrida, Arnhem Land, and similar numbers at Yalata, South Australia, and on numerous other Aboriginal settlements, have "inadequate" parents in such abundance. Indeed, recent experience with outstation communities reveals that strong sanctions against alcohol can exist (Morice, 1976). This suggests that an important factor in the *apparent* abnegation of parental responsibility or concern for petrol-sniffing may relate to the amount of control the parents are allowed to exercise over their own lives.

Stryde (1977 : 57) points out in his survey of Indian settlements in Canada, that writers usually cite one causative factor to the exclusion of all others: either poverty, lack of recreation, poor education, irresponsibility, parental alcoholism, cultural disintegration, acculturation or stress, for example. The findings of such studies as that by Kaufman of Pueblo Indians should not be forgotten either. Kaufman (1973 : 1063) found that although the incidence of broken homes and alcoholism in the community was high, it was no higher in the home life of children who had sniffed than in those who had not.

One problem of accepting a "deprived" family background as an explanation for behaviour such as petrol-sniffing, is that it may be yet another instance of "blaming the victim". Colin Tatz (1972 : 5), at a national seminar on Aboriginal Health Services in 1972, spoke on welfare bureaucracies who saw

> causality and culpability . . . in the "transients" at Amoonguna or the "immigrant Pintubi" at Papunya . . . The Aboriginal penchant for grog, their stubborn adherence to what is seen to be a "bad" traditional way of life, their general perversity in refusing or rejecting enlightenment and, worse, their ingratitude, are clearly at work . . . Causality, in short, lies in *their* culture, customs and cussedness.

Another group of commentaries on petrol-sniffing have stressed its role of tension-release or stimulus-seeking (Collins, 1978; Nurcombe *et al.*, 1970 : 369), which reflect boredom and the lack of other means of relieving that boredom. But "boredom" itself is a term disguising a wealth of experiences that stream in upon the Aboriginal child from all sides. These experiences are seen by some observers to be related to structural and socio-political factors, such as the loss of land and the consequent social and cultural disruption (Sargent, 1978 : 6). Eastwell (1979 : 223) documents such a case at Maningrida in Arnhem Land, where petrol-sniffing was prevalent among the children of four "deprived" clans, who in 1978 were the only clans lacking outstations. Prompted by the "problems of inhaling", the Gunavidji and the Nakara clans began to make efforts to move out of the settlement on to outstations, although this would mean relinquishing their influence on the settlement council. The movement to decentralize communities and for smaller family groups to live once more on their homelands in some cases has acted as a curb on petrol-sniffing. Eastwell suggests that it is "uniquely a problem of the new towns". However, sniffing *is* apparent, even on some of the Pitjantjatjara homelands settlements in the north-west of South Australia, despite the decentralized nature of these communities.

Tomlinson (1975 : 76) comments that Groote Eylandt children do not sniff petrol, and suggests that this is because of the strong clan leadership and consciousness by the people of their separateness. He points also to the necessity for control of settlements to be handed over to Aboriginal residents. On missions and settlements all over Australia, Europeans still control firmly the decision-making and organizational work of the towns.

A WIDER PERSPECTIVE

In order to highlight the extent to which many Aboriginal people have been encroached upon and systematically removed farther and farther from their original territory, a description of a South Australian community is offered. The Pitjantjatjara people who now live at Yalata, 1000 kilometres west of Adelaide on the edge of the Nullarbor Plain, number approximately 400, of whom 104 were between the ages of five and fifteen in 1977. Over the last two years particularly, the community has experienced a rapid upsurge in petrol-sniffing in this age group, along with court appearances for juvenile offences by 75 per cent of the sixteen- to eighteen-year-old males.

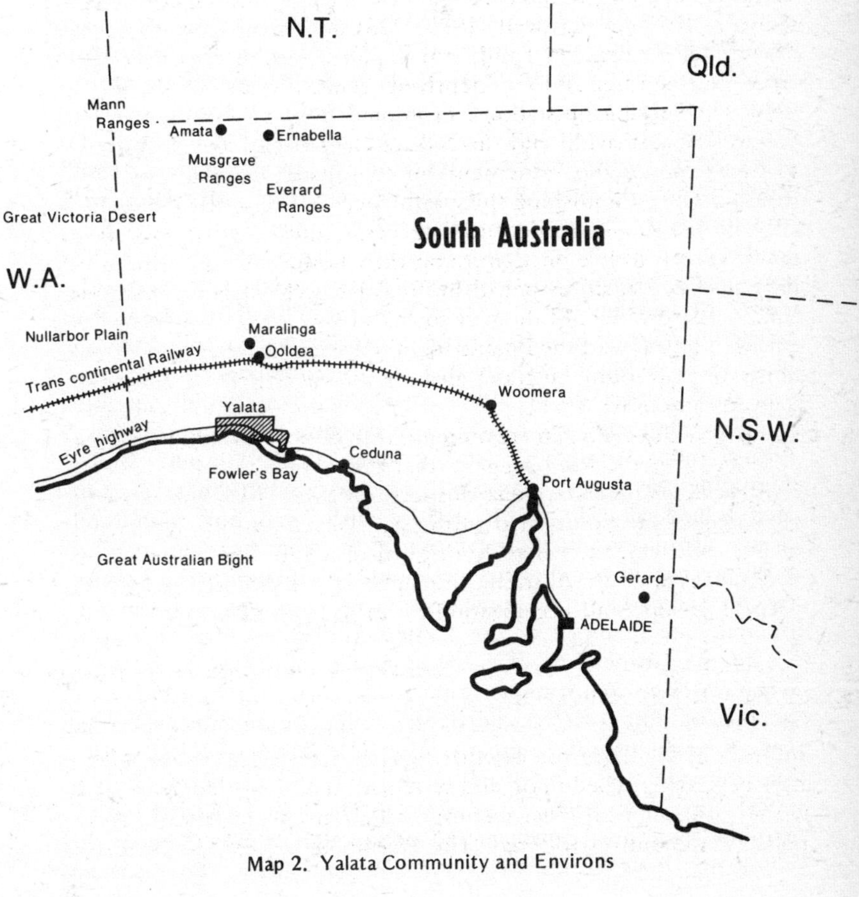

Map 2. Yalata Community and Environs

The Yalata estate is not the traditional homeland of the people who are now settled on it. The people came from the "spinifex" — the Great Victoria Desert region and the Mann, Musgrave and Everard Ranges in the north of South Australia (Berndt, 1941). Their traditional routes had brought them regularly to visit Ooldea Soak, a permanent source of water on the northern fringe of the Nullarbor Plain, which became a water supply for the building of the Trans-Australia railway-line between 1912 and 1917. During the building of the railway, with the creation of sidings, camps and ration depots, Aboriginal people were drawn to the area by the activity and the source of food, and hundreds of people arrived to camp along the line. In 1919, Mrs Daisy Bates set up her camp on the sand-dunes overlooking Ooldea Soak, in order to help the Aboriginal people by treating them with her "grandmotherly remedies" and by sharing her food. In 1933, a pioneer woman missionary arrived representing the United Aborigines Mission, and within two months she was being issued with rations and medicines for "infirm natives" by the Office of the Chief Protector of Aborigines. This was a dramatic concession on the part of the government to the work of the mission (which was, and is, an evangelical "faith" mission), and constituted an unspoken rebuttal to Mrs Bates, who had constantly requested this kind of aid herself.

When the railway was built, the Aboriginal people utilized it for transport to ceremonies in Western Australia, and the "Kalgoorlie mobs" likewise travelled to Ooldea on the train. The missionaries were not happy about the flow of Aborigines to and from the west, because this constantly depleted the numbers in their boys' and girls' homes. On the other hand, when large groups attended Ooldea ceremonies, the missionaries saw this as an opportunity to "reach" more Aborigines "with the sound of the Gospel" (United Aborigines *Messenger*, 1 May 1952). The mission buildings were situated in the soak itself, and by 1950 a church hall, houses and children's dormitories (to house those taken from their parents) had been erected. Physical drill, boys' brigades (mending and knitting for the girls), Christian endeavour, daily morning prayers were offered. The ideology of the United Aborigines Mission was to "instil the Gospel into the Aborigines if they were approached when children ... if tribal customs could be broken down, and the people could be induced to drop their superstition and cruel tribal laws, their lot would be greatly improved" (*Messenger*, 1929). The Superintendent was reported by Ronald and Catherine Berndt (1951 : 137), who worked at Ooldea in 1939–40, as having photographed ceremonial *tjuringas* and deliberately shown them to the uninitiated boys. In the magazine *Messenger*, there were constant references to the difficulties faced by those Aborigines who had embraced Christianity and yet were in a native camp, surrounded by subtle, sinister and Satanic influences.

Despite the fervour of missionary activity, living conditions at Ooldea were far from comfortable. There were frequent dust-storms and the buildings were constantly in danger of sinking into sand-drifts. The South Australian government began to look for an alternative reserve for the Aboriginal people more urgently, because the British were planning to test atomic weapons at Emu Field, some distance to the north. They later chose another test-site, near to the supply-base of the railway. This was Maralinga, only forty kilometres north of Ooldea Soak. Ooldea was to be closed down, and the people transported even further south, almost to the coast, to a new reserve. In March 1951, the government purchased the leases of 4560 square kilometres held by the Yalata Pastoral Company, a tract of land south of the Trans-Australia railway-line, at the head of the Great Australian Bight, with a poor water supply and hard, salty ground. The original lease included the old Yalata homestead, near Fowler's Bay, and its accompanying more fertile farming land, but when some local farmers complained that "good farmland" was to be used for an Aboriginal reserve (Hampel, 1977 : 2), this part of the property was deliberately omitted from the final lease.

There had been an ongoing dispute between the Lutheran Church, which controlled other missions in the southern area, and the United Aborigines Mission, over which of them was to carry on the mission work with the Ooldea people. United Aborigines Missionary, Harrie Green, wrote in the *Messenger*:

> The powers of evil are against us . . . are coming out more strongly than ever to stop us from going and caring for our people. Pray God will fight for us and give us strength.

At a crucial stage in the negotiations, an internal division split the federal and local United Aborigines Missions, and their future in the area become untenable. When Yalata opened in 1952, it was under the aegis of the Lutheran Church.

The winding-up process at Ooldea was chaotic. The Chief Protector was worried that the fifty boys and girls in the Ooldea Children's Home might fall "into the hands of the camp natives" (Hampel, 1977 : 7) — many of whom, it is worth pointing out, would have been their parents. A deputation of Lutherans arrived to transport the people south. But as one pastor wrote (Hampel, 1977 : 8)

> Most of the Aboriginal people were not willing to move south to the Fowlers Bay area, but to the north and west. They took their children with them. Only six children were brought . . .

and another

> to [the missionaries'] disappointment they discovered that only about twenty per cent of the natives were willing to travel southward; the majority wanted to go to Ernabella or Western Australia. What prompted them to do this we have not been able to determine as yet.

One group did in fact set off for Ernabella, and reached Tarcoola, but inexplicably returned some weeks later and were brought down to Yalata.[4]

Aided by the Woomera patrol officer, whose task it had been to clear the test-site of "natives", small groups of people were trucked down to the new reserve. The first task of their new spiritual overseers was to distribute sweets and tobacco, before assembling the people for (Lutheran) prayers.

THE PRESENT CONTEXT

At the official handover of responsibility, the Lutheran Church undertook that: "the younger men will be trained to look after the property, and the children will be educated and trained to take over the station in the years ahead" (Hampel, 1977 : 22). Twenty-six years later, the running of the settlement, with its sheep-station, roadhouse (providing petrol to travellers on the Eyre Highway and, inadvertently, to the community's sniffers), store, school, clinic and workshop, still is entirely in the hands of European staff (who by 1977, had increased in number from sixteen to forty-nine). However, a recently (1980) instituted pre-employment training scheme by the Department of Further Education is undertaking to train Aboriginal assistants to work with white supervisors in various roles in the settlement. The scheme is confronting some difficulty with settlement staff, who suspect that their jobs might be taken over, and Aboriginal trainees have been told that they are getting "too big for their boots".

The young boys of the community are frequently in trouble with the local police, whose car is a regular sight on the settlement, mainly on charges of breaking, entering and stealing. Their items of choice seem to be predominantly useful ones: food, soft drinks and sleeping bags. The electric stoves of the school domestic science unit are sometimes used to cook stolen food. The prime targets for breaking and entering are the school, private homes and the community store. Although the store's profits are supposedly fed back into the "community", and although it "belongs" to the community, evidently it is not perceived by Aborigines as being "theirs".

Another community enterprise over which it has little direct control is the roadhouse on the main highway, three kilometres south of the settlement. The roadhouse is constructed with building materials from the deserted Maralinga Village, headquarters of the atomic testing in the 1950s, to which Yalata was given the salvage rights. At the present time, although "owned" by the community, it is operated by Europeans, both at the pumps, behind the snack-bar and in the dining-room (the only non-white employee being a part-Aboriginal man from Ceduna, the nearest town), and this has been the cause of much grumbling and resentment among the people. Aboriginal men from Yalata, however, were employed as labourers to demolish the buildings at Maralinga. This had its advantages, from the perspective of the ex-pastor of the settlement: he thought the community gained much in every way from the salvaging: many people found "gainful employment and a change of scenery, working on the Maralinga project" (Hampel, 1977 : 39).

The Maralinga story continues, however, for since 1976, there has been a series of public outcries over the burial of radioactive waste on the site; the level of contamination, which will last for another fifty years (Adelaide *Advertiser*, 16 October 1979), and the revelation that many deaths from cancer have occurred among ex-military and civilian personnel employed during the seven atomic tests carried out in 1956 and 1957. More recently (April 1980), the concern has extended to the Aboriginal people, some of whom after the closure of Ooldea Mission would have inevitably eluded the army patrols, and consequently remained in the test area. One such family, who now live at Yalata emerged from the prohibited zone in 1957 and had to be showered in a decontamination caravan because of their high level of body radiation (*Advertiser*, 16 April 1980). Along with other Aboriginal people suspected of contamination, this family waited six months for the promised Health Commission medical checkup. This unfortunate aftermath contributes yet another factor of unease to the present circumstances of the Yalata community.

Another common offence is illegal use of vehicles, an activity that has become more prevalent since the white residents this year (1980) have fitted burglar alarms to all major buildings and homes in the settlement. Panel vans are the most desired vehicles, since they allow more storage space for people and supplies, and often quite young boys will travel long distances outback before they are caught. When vehicles are taken in an organized way, along with petrol and supplies of food, they are always driven *north*, towards the Pitjantjatjara homelands, away from the towns of the white-dominated south, and away from Yalata.

The relationship between such "offending" behaviour and petrol-sniffing is difficult to establish firmly, for at Yalata, the young people who get caught, and who end up in the Children's Court, are an older age group than those who sniff petrol regularly. Sniffers can range from age seven to, in some communities, those in their early twenties (Nurcombe, 1974 : 67). Another major distinction is that at Yalata, girls participate in sniffing, but do not show up in the court statistics. It may be that they do not actually commit so many offences, or alternatively, the white authorities may be more lenient in reporting them.

On at least one occasion, an outbreak of petrol-sniffing in the community has been linked to discord within the white settlement. It occurred after the sacking of a staff member, which precipitated much intrigue and factionalism in the community.

RESISTANCE: OVERT AND COVERT

Sniffing may take place during the school lunchbreak, at evening film-showings, or at any time. A popular venue is the schoolyard or an empty backyard. (The school principal's is popular.)

Defying the school and all that it stands for (in the form of order, adults, European society) by sniffing within its precincts, is just one overt form of the rebellion that sniffing may symbolically represent. The school, usually the largest physical presence on a settlement, is perhaps also the institution with most psychological impact: it "places enormous pressures on the child to conform, to compete, to 'make progress' ... measured by European concepts and traditions" (Sargent, 1978 : 3). When teachers are asked about petrol-sniffing, their perspective is inevitably that of its effects on the quality of performance. Teachers on Elcho Island described the bulk of petrol-sniffers as being "non-achievers" (Tomlinson, 1975 : 74), and teachers at Yalata said some children had "gone downhill" since they began sniffing. One headteacher remarked, revealingly, that there were "more sniffers on the school premises at midnight than there are at midday" (Eastwell, 1979 : 222).

There are accounts from elsewhere in Australia of children apparently trying to prove their invulnerability to spirits by going into graveyards while "sniffed up" (Tomlinson, 1975 : 75). Children also tell of "travelling around" and visiting other places when they hallucinate. Sniffing hallucinations offer exciting and frightening experiences of being chased, or shot at; of the ground opening up to swallow the sniffer; of hearing Rod Stewart singing; hunting wombats, and of having sex or watching others do so.[5] Petrol-sniffing allows a certain diminished responsibility for one's actions. This in turn makes breaking the law easier, and permits acting-up in front of adults. Such defiance parallels the explanation of getting drunk at Yalata, which is frequently offered by Aboriginal people: that when they drink they "get strength" to say what they really think, and to say these things to white people. It is certainly illustrative of a community's perception of its power (or lack of it) that adults do not feel able to speak up on their own behalf or criticize without the support of drink.

On a covert level, the sheer intractability of the sniffers, who seem untouched by rational attempts to educate them about the harmful effects of petrol-sniffing (attempts usually instituted by concerned adults and nursing sisters), constitutes a form of passive resistance in itself. The consistent disregard for the dangers, and in some cases the public flaunting of the behaviour, also are indicative of a form of defiance documented by Robertson (1970 : 8) in her work on Indian reservations in Canada. She suggests that the "real" resistance lies in the instinctive gearing of reserve society to alienate white people as much as possible.

INTERVENTION STRATEGIES

Faced with the immediacy of the situation in the day-to-day existence of a community, many of the solutions that have been suggested have been punitive, limited in vision or diversionary. For example, many communities have instituted extra recreational activities after school ("prime crime time"), in an attempt to deflect sniffers from their activities. However, often sniffers are the very children who do not attend such activities anyway. That such facilities are sorely needed by some communities, there is no doubt: at Amata, for instance, the pool-table, which is ostensibly for the use of the young boys after school, is constantly taken over by older men. The quality of staff (if they are outsiders) involved in such ventures and the degree of rapport with the people must play a significant part in the success or failure of the programme. Papunya, in the Northern Territory, under the auspices of the Y.M.C.A. set up committees that endeavoured to "de-isolate the individuals concerned by deliberately including them in conversations, games and activities" (Dalton-Morgan, 1978 : 33). However, it appears that the committees operated successfully only during the tenure of the Y.M.C.A. officer concerned, and they have now ceased. But this is not to deny that some chronic sniffers may benefit from some form of individualized therapy.

Punishment by relatives seems merely to increase the resentment towards authority figures, and Sargent (1978 : 5) comments that sniffing could flourish as a result. The effect is self-perpetuating, in that the child stays with his companions rather than goes home. Other communities have tried shaming the sniffers and their parents by publicly exhibiting lists of names, and banning them from using the community's services. Some children have been banished to outlying camps for sniffing-related offences, but are often received as "minor heroes" on their return (Eastwell, 1979 : 223).

Bremer Island, off the coast of Nhulunbuy (Gove), was used as a detention centre for Aboriginal children; it lacked the status and comforts of a city or prison placement for children in trouble. However, sniffing continued within the nearby settlement, Yirrkala, despite a decrease in "criminal behaviour" (Sargent, 1978 : 7). The scheme caused some controversy and due to lack of government commitment, it has been discontinued. The children often recommence sniffing when they return home, which is hardly surprising. Even when communities lock up their petrol supplies, petrol tanks and wrecked vehicles, the ingenuity of the sniffers seems to win out.

Education about the physical dangers of sniffing apparently is not sufficient *in itself* as a deterrent. This is certainly borne out in the case of the glue-sniffing epidemic in the United States which was *spread* by exposure of its dangerous, even fatal outcome (Brecher *et al.*, 1972).

In his Canadian study, Stryde (1977 : 45–52) concludes that there is no "blanket" formula for curbing sniffing. He emphasizes the uniqueness of each community and its context, the rapport that may or may not exist between white medical personnel and the people, and the degree of involvement of local people in decision-making and implementation.

It seems that the framework of dependency that began at Ooldea Soak has its present-day echo in the prominence of Europeans in all aspects of the daily running of the Yalata community, and in the capacity of the Aboriginal people to have allowed that prominence to occur. People will give their individual suggestions as to the reasons for petrol-sniffing — the "grog", the bad films shown to children, the lack of an on-the-spot policeman. But a thoughtful staff member suggested that the community and the Europeans needed to sit down and take a long, hard look at how things were organized: "Everything else is just a band-aid."

CONCLUSION: THE HUMAN MATRIX

We have examined some of the approaches taken by investigators when attempting to understand petrol-sniffing among Aboriginal children and located this problem in its socio-historical context for one community.

Although people in authority express concern about the medical consequences of petrol-sniffing, much of the literature betrays a concern with order, "disrespect" and discipline; with the smooth running (at all costs) of the settlement; and even with the quantity and type of sexual activity that adolescents may indulge in: all this under the heading of fears about petrol-sniffing. Terms such as "illicit" and phrases such as "children were *apprehended*" abound, and the major "disorders" that are said to result from sniffing behaviour seem to be the defiance of authority and "anti-social" behaviour. These essentially are judgements based on European notions of what constitutes "deviant behaviour". Such judgements do not greatly help communities or health personnel to dissect out what is *really* harmful in petrol-sniffing or to appreciate the wider social matrix in which it occurs.

The helpfulness or otherwise of all European advisors and employees must lie in their ability to *listen*, their rapport with the people, and the extent to which Aboriginal people themselves feel involved in whatever programmes they implement. Aborigines also have a right to know about the effects of petrol and lead on the body, how to watch for signs of neurological damage and to know of the steps taken by other communities in Australia. But if education is to be a role taken by Europeans, it must be education of a special kind, a variant of Freire's (1972) "problem-posing education", in which people are encouraged to think critically about their past and present circumstances and to understand the structural determinants of social events (Freire, 1978).

Petrol-sniffing is a behaviour that defies "cures" by medical science, either before or after the damage is done. Whatever the community's attempts to intervene might be, its power to evoke a feeling of strength — so that demands can be made, decision-making democratized and ideas tried out fully and patiently — will form the basis of any change in the behaviour of the young.

ACKNOWLEDGEMENTS

A grant from the Criminology Research Council has made part of this research possible, through the Department of Psychiatry, School of Medicine, Flinders University of South Australia. The Head of Department, Professor Ross Kalucy, has been generous in his support for this work.

We would like to thank Aboriginal and white friends at Yalata for their assistance; and Dr Janice Reid, Dr Lee Sackett, Dr Jeff Collman and Peter Bishop for their comments on an earlier draft of this paper. Also we wish to thank Ms Helen Swift, Research Assistant in the Department of Psychiatry, who painstakingly compiled data on the effects of lead on the human body, and from whose compilation we have drawn.

NOTES

[1] The first known accounts (according to Brecher *et al.*, 1972) were from Arizona and Colorado in 1959; two Denver reporters investigated and their newspaper story in August 1959 carried the headline "Some Glues are Dangerous: Heavy Inhalation Can Cause Anaemia or Brain Damage". It explained how to sniff glue and what its effects were. Six to eight months later, the Denver police reported they had investigated some fifty cases of glue-sniffing. More scare newspaper reports followed in 1960, and in 1961 Denver police arrested 282 juveniles for sniffing.

[2] The media in the early 1960s were full of reports of deaths due to glue-sniffing; however, when these were tracked down, it was found that nine alleged deaths had each been reported many times and that six of these were not due to glue fumes but to asphyxiation from the plastic bags used (Brecher *et al.*, 1972). One death was reported from petrol-sniffing on an Aboriginal reserve at Gerard in South Australia, in March 1979; another occurred at Amata in 1976.

[3] The *National Times* of 14–19 November 1977 (p. 49) published a sensational article entitled: "Grog and Petrol Sniffing", which stated unequivocally: "once well under, the sniffer needs food and excitement, and gets both by breaking into somebody's home".

[4] It has been suggested that "totem boards and sacred regalia" had been hidden north of Tarcoola and that the men wanted to retrieve them (Hampel, 1977 : 11).

[5] These descriptions were given by Yalata children to Geoff Rogers, to whom we are grateful.

REFERENCES

Bass M., 1970. "Sudden Sniffing Death", *Journal of the American Medical Association* 12, no. 2 : 2075–79.

——, 1978. "Death from Sniffing Gasoline", *New England Journal of Medicine* 299, no. 4 : 203.

Beattie, A. D., Moore, M. R., and Goldberg, A., 1972. "Tetra-ethyl Lead Poisoning", *Lancet* (1 July) : 12–15.

Beckett, J., 1964. "Aborigines, Alcohol and Assimilation", in *Aborigines Now*, ed. M. Reay (Sydney : Angus & Robertson), pp. 32–47.

Berndt, R. M., 1941. "Tribal Migrations and Myths Centring on Ooldea, S.A.", *Oceania* 12, no. 1 : 1–20.

—— and Berndt, C. H., 1951. *From Black to White in South Australia* (Melbourne : Cheshire).

Black, P. D., 1967. "Mental Illness due to the Voluntary Inhalation of Petrol Vapour", *Medical Journal of Australia* 2 : 70–71.

Boeckx, R. L., Postl, B., and Coodin, F. J., 1977. "Gasoline Sniffing and Tetra-ethyl Lead Poisoning in Children", *Pediatrics* 60 (August) : 140–45.

Brecher, E. M., *et al.*, 1972. "How to Launch a Nationwide Drug Menace", in *Licit and Illicit Drugs* (Boston : Little Brown), pp. 321–34.

Cernkovitch, S. A., 1978. "Conceptual and Empirical Ambiguity in Class-oriented Theories of Crime and Delinquency", *International Journal of Criminology and Penology* 6 : 105–20.

Collins, D., 1978. On petrol-sniffing, in Northern Territory. Legislative Assembly, *Debates* (28 February–9 March) : 697–700.

Dalton-Morgan, D., 1978. "Petrol Sniffing: Papunya . . . a Community Solution", *Forum* (Australian Crime Prevention Council Quarterly Journal) 1, no. 1 : 32–33.

Eastwell, H. D., 1979. "Petrol Inhalation in Aboriginal Towns: Its Remedy, the Homelands Movement", *Medical Journal of Australia* 2 : 221–24.

Freire, P., 1972. *Pedagogy of the Oppressed* (Harmondsworth : Penguin).

———, 1978. *Pedagogy in Process: The Letters to Guinea-Bisseau* (London: Writers & Readers).

Garnys, V. P., Freeman, R., and Smythe, L. E., 1979. *Lead Burden of Sydney Schoolchildren* (Sydney : University of New South Wales Publication. 400 p.).

Gold, N., 1963. "Self Intoxication by Petrol Vapour Inhalation", *Medical Journal of Australia* 2 : 582–84.

Hampel, N. A., 1977. *Yalata Lutheran Mission, 1952–1977* (Yalata, S.A.).

Hetzel, B. S., 1975. "Religion and Change in an Age of Social Change", in *Cultures in Collision*, ed. I. Pilowsky (Adelaide : Australian National Association for Mental Health), pp. 274–81.

Huey, R., 1978. "Petrol Sniffing in Traditional Communities" (unpublished report. Mimeo. Dept. Aboriginal Affairs files, Canberra).

Jager, M., 1975. "Native Children Sniffing Gasoline", *The Journal* (Addiction Research Foundation, Ontario) 4, no. 1 (July) : 1.

Kaufman, A., 1973. "Gasoline Sniffing among Children in a Pueblo Indian Village", *Pediatrics* 51, no. 6 : 1060–64.

MacAndrew, C., and Edgerton, R. B., 1970. *Drunken Comportment: A Social Explanation* (Chicago : Aldine).

Matza, D., 1969. *Becoming Deviant* (Englewood Cliffs, N.J. : Prentice-Hall).

Morice, R. D., 1976. "Woman Dancing Dreaming: Psychosocial Benefits of the Aboriginal Outstation Movement", *Medical Journal of Australia* 2 : 939–42.

Needleman, H. L., *et al.*, 1979. "Deficits in Psychologic and Classroom Performance of Children with Elevated Dentine Lead Levels", *New England Journal of Medicine* 300, no. 13 : 689–95.

Nurcombe, B., 1974. "Petrol Inhalation in Arnhem Land", in *Better Health for Aborigines? A Report of a National Seminar at Monash University*, ed. B. S. Hetzel (St Lucia : Queensland University Press), pp. 66–71.

———, Bianchi, G., Money, J., and Cawte, J., 1970. "A Hunger for Stimuli:

The Psychosocial Background of Petrol Inhalation", *British Journal of Medical Psychology* 43 : 367–74.

Robertson, H., 1970. *Reservations Are For Indians* (Toronto : Lewis & Samuel).

Sargent, G., 1978. "Petrol Sniffing in East Arnhem Land: A Resumé" (unpublished report from Welfare Officer, Nhulunbuy, N.T.), pp. 1–9. Dept. Aboriginal Affairs files, Canberra.

Schmitt, R. C., and Abston, S., 1972. "Gasoline Sniffing in Children Leading to Severe Burn Injury", *Journal of Paediatrics* 80 (June) : 1021–23.

Stryde, W., 1977. "A Report on Gasoline Sniffing in Manitoba" (unpublished), 15 August. The Non-medical Use of Drugs Directorate, Health Protection Branch, Dept. National Health and Welfare and Alcoholism Foundation of Manitoba.

Tatz, C., 1972. "The Politics of Aboriginal Health: Paper given at National Seminar on Aboriginal Health, Monash University, 15–17 May", *Politics* 7, no. 2 (November) : 3–23.

Tomlinson, J. R., 1975. "Petrol Sniffing in the Northern Territory", *Australian Journal of Alcohol and Drug Dependence* 2, no. 3 : 74–77.

Valpey, R., Sumi, S. M., Copass, M. K., and Gobie, G. J., 1978. "Acute and Chronic Progressive Encephalopathy due to Gasoline Sniffing", *Neurology* (May) : 507–10.

Watson, J. M., 1978. "Clinical and Laboratory Investigations in 132 Cases of Solvent Abuse", *Medical Science Law* 18, no. 1 : 40–43.

Webber, D. L., 1976. "Petrol Inhalation and Social Dislocation in Arnhem Land", in *Report* of National Alcohol and Drug Dependency, Multidisciplinary Institute, Canberra pp. 139–41.

Part Two

Medicine and Health: The Traditional Systems

Sickness is a universal human experience. In response to the threat that it poses to the well-being of the individual and integrity of the group, all societies have developed techniques of prevention and treatment. Aboriginal societies, no less than those elsewhere, possess strategies designed to minimize injury and illness. Prevention has many faces, and Aboriginal concepts of prevention vary from place to place. At the physical level, it can include seeking protection from the cold, wind or rain, eating a fresh diet of both flesh and vegetable foods, maintaining a balanced emotional state, and exercising and sleeping sufficiently to maintain bodily well-being. At a more inclusive level, prevention encompasses personal relationships and religious injunctions. Efforts to avoid sickness are based on laws governing behaviour. Preventive measures can include avoiding foods prohibited during ceremonies or life crises, obeying ritual proscriptions, taking care not to abuse one's land or trespass on the territories of others, avoiding prohibited sacred sites or approaching them with ritual protection, observing debts and obligations to others, containing anger, violence or jealousy, exercising caution in interactions with strangers, and taking steps to avoid sorcery or open conflict with others.

When individuals become ill they, or their relatives, can draw on their community's repertoire of medical skills and treatments. Aboriginal medical resources include herbal medicines, diet, external remedies such as ochre, smoke, steam and heat, the skills of the healer, and, if the affliction is thought to have an interpersonal or spiritual aetiology, procedures for restoring harmony. The Aboriginal approach to both prophylaxis and curing is a holistic one. It recognizes the physical, personal and spiritual dimension of life and health. In many ways, the Aboriginal perspective on health and illness is closer than that of Western medicine to the World Health Organization's definition of health — "a state of complete physical, mental and social well-being and not merely the absence of disease or infirmity".

The chapters in this section explore in detail Aboriginal views of health and the traditional therapeutic repertoires utilized in times of illness. The first chapter, "Ten Fish for One Man: Some Anbarra Attitudes towards Food and Health" by Betty Meehan, describes the attitudes of the Anbarra of north-central Arnhem Land to the foods that their land provides. One does not need a knowledge of the scientific literature to be aware of the changes in Aboriginal nutrition wrought by the shift from an independent, semi-nomadic lifestyle to a dependent, sedentary one. A people who once drew upon a natural larder of food now subsist, in most large communities, on processed, packaged foods, particularly on cheap and durable items such as tea, damper and tinned meat. This diet, high in carbohydrate and low in protein, vitamins and minerals, fosters deficiency diseases, diabetes, obesity and cardiovascular disease.

Why do Aborigines eat so poorly? Do they understand our notion of a balanced diet? Many efforts at nutrition education have been based on the assumption that they do not. The "they-don't-know-what's-good-for-them" philosophy is implicit in the approach of many service agencies to Aborigines, but particularly prominent in much of the dietary instruction given in schools and "home management" programmes. Meehan, who has conducted fieldwork in Arnhem Land since 1958, provides ample evidence that disregard for the balance, quality or freshness of food is not a primary cause of nutritional imbalance. She describes, in succulent detail, the wealth and nutritional values of sea and land species and of plant foods that constitute the diet of Anbarra living at their outstation, the variety of their cooking techniques, the pride in preparation and the selectivity among foods of differing ages and attributes. When they are living on their land, the Anbarra not only hunt like lords on their own estates, but enjoy a diet that would satisfy nutritionist and gourmet alike.

In the chapter "Sickness and Health in Western Arnhem Land: A Traditional Perspective", Catherine Berndt, who has worked in western Arnhem Land since the 1940s, selects certain of the myths of the people to explain their concept of the relationship between health and land, religion and social relationships. The Aboriginal universe, as Berndt shows, is peopled with spirits, major creative figures and mythical beings whose words and exploits provide the bases of the moral, religious and practical codes of human behaviour. Berndt's chapter is particularly relevant today, for it deals with an area of Australia that has been, and continues to be, an arena of keen dispute between mining companies, government and Aborigines about the valuable minerals on their land. Arnhem Land has seen two notable conflicts over the land and its wealth. In 1971, the

Yolngu people of north-eastern Arnhem Land recognized the threat to their land of a proposed bauxite mining operation and went to the Australian courts to fight for legal recognition of their land ownership. In this celebrated case (*Milirrpum and Others* v. *Nabalco Pty Ltd and the Commonwealth of Australia* (1971)), they and their counsel presented overwhelming evidence to validate their rights of occupation and inheritance: recognized boundaries, myths of possession, ancient rituals and sacred paintings. Though they lost this case, they, with the people of western and central Arnhem Land, were given freehold title to their land several years later under the *Land Rights Act (Northern Territory)* 1976. For the people of Oenpelli, who were facing the prospect of large-scale uranium mining, the Act was a doubtful asset. They now had title to their land, but no right to refuse mining: only the right to negotiate. By the end of the decade, the excavation of uranium on their land had begun.

The Aborigines of Arnhem Land, as Berndt shows, view the events of the recent and distant past as material to the present; for them, health is the outcome of the social and spiritual well-being of each clan. Incursions into this well-being are incursions into health. At one time, these incursions — religious and social breaches of the law — could be managed by the intervention of traditional healers and ritual specialists, or by members and heads of families. Today their control is limited, for many offences against law and land are committed by Europeans. As Aborigines have predicted, the outcome of these disruptions is often sickness and social conflict.

David Biernoff's chapter, "Psychiatric and Anthropological Interpretations of 'Aberrant' Behaviour in an Aboriginal Community", is based on his work at Numbulwar, a settlement in south-eastern Arnhem Land. His study introduces some critical issues, which can only be touched upon here yet require some introduction. In Australia, there exists a substantial body of literature on the psychiatric morbidity and psychological characteristics of Australian Aborigines. Some of these studies have provoked concern on the part of social scientists. Among other things, social scientists have criticized the inadequate periods of field research on which they are based and the underlying assumptions that psychiatric categories are valid cross-culturally.[1] They have also questioned the largely undocumented assertions that Aboriginal societies show a good deal of "endogenous", culturally-determined pathology. The more responsible of these studies lend themselves to scholarly argument. The less responsible are often superficial, scientifically unsound and grossly ethnocentric.[2]

This is not to say that "mental disorders" cannot exist in Aboriginal societies. It seems very likely that a small number of people in every human community are unusually disturbed, frightened or confused, or in some way "abnormal" in the way they think or feel. Beyond recognizing these people, or having them pointed out by members of their families or communities, the question arises as to what a Western-trained health worker should do. Is it necessary to understand the world view of a society in order to help its "disturbed" members? Can Western eyes understand the reality of another culture at all? Is it legitimate to apply psychiatric labels developed in the Western medical tradition to other societies? What place should drugs, personal therapy or institutionalization have in the treatment of these people? Should the disturbed person's treatment and rehabilitation be the responsibility of his or her community? How can health workers support the family and help them foster a therapeutic milieu? Are Aboriginal mental health workers the answer, and if so, whose model of psychiatric care should they hold — the Western or the Aboriginal? These are just a few of the questions that are crucial to the pursuit of psychiatric work in any cultural context. They are particularly relevant when the culture is alien to the doctor, nurse or health worker responsible for a community's health services. At the moment, all are urgently in need of sound research.

Biernoff demonstrates the value of such research in his discussion of the cultural context in which mental "aberrations" are played out. He shows that Aboriginal concepts of mental health are tightly enmeshed with the spiritual identity of the individual and his or her family, and that this identity is ultimately derived from the land of his or her birth. All serious sickness flows from crises in human and spiritual relationships, and these often relate to the use (or misuse) of land. Biernoff argues that few, if any, of the psychological and psychiatric studies among Aborigines have focused on the conceptual models that Aboriginal people utilize to explain "abnormal" behaviour. A lack of such cross-cultural awareness limits the health practitioner's ability to relate to the patient or to alleviate — let alone cure — his condition.

The final chapter in this section describes natural curing resources used by members of a community in the tropical north. " 'Bush Medicines': The Pharmacopoeia of the Yolngu of Arnhem Land", deals with the medicinal plants of the people of north-eastern Arnhem Land. Neville Scarlett, a botanist, Neville White, a biological anthropologist, and Janice Reid, a medical anthropologist, have pooled their knowledge of Yolngu bush medicines to describe the pharmacopoeia of the Yolngu and its use today. The authors have identified over a hundred bush medicines, each with its own mode of preparation, indications and method of administration. The medicinal plants are presented under their botanical and Aboriginal names, and categorized in terms of the conditions for which they are used. Their historical roots and their place in the wider medical system are also discussed.

Systematic studies of Aboriginal medicines are few and scattered. Analyses of the active constituents of plant medicines, such as those carried out by pharmacologists for some South American plants and Asian medicines, have yet to be initiated on any scale in Australia. The day when new and valuable drugs may be isolated from Aboriginal medicines and added to the corpus of Western medical knowledge is still a long way off. In the meantime, Aborigines continue to prepare and use their own "bush medicines", transmitting this knowledge both to their children and to researchers interested in learning about these natural resources.

NOTES

1 For a critique of this assumption, see A. J. Marsella, "Madness and Culture: Exporting the Cuckoo's Nest" (an interview with Marsella), *East West Perspectives* (East West Centre, Honolulu, Ha.) 1, no. 3 (1980) : 30–36.

2 Perhaps the most notable example of the second of these categories is a study carried out by Arthur Hippler on culture and personality among the Yolngu of Arnhem Land. (See A. Hippler, "Culture and Personality Perspective of the Yolngu of Northeastern Arnhem Land: Part 1 — Early Socialization", *Journal of Psychological Anthropology* 1, no. 2 (1978) : 221–44.) This paper is suffused with an ideology of the inferiority of Aboriginal culture and portrays one Arnhem Land community as ridden by socialized, and collective, personality disorders. When the paper appeared (in a journal founded and edited by Hippler), it was condemned on professional and ethical grounds by such bodies as the Australian Institute of Aboriginal Studies and by members of the Australian academic community, including cross-cultural psychologists and anthropologists with extensive research experience in Yolngu communities. (See, for instance, Annette Hamilton, "A Comment on Arthur Hippler's Paper, 'Culture and Personality Perspective of the Yolngu of Northeastern Arnhem Land: Part 1' . . .", *Mankind* 12, no. 2 (1979) : 164–69; Joseph Reser, "Australian Aboriginal Man's Inhumanity to Man: A Case of Cultural Distortion", *American Anthropologist* 83, no. 2 (1981) : 387–93; and J. P. Reser, G. E. Kearney and B. Drinkwater, "Cultural Singularism: Or Who Wears the Blinkers", *IACCP Cross-cultural Psychology Newsletter* 14, no. 5 (1980) : 1–6).

5
Ten Fish for One Man: Some Anbarra Attitudes towards Food and Health

Betty Meehan

During the 1973 wet season at Lalarr-gadjirripa, an Aboriginal outstation on the northern coast of Arnhem Land, as the camp was consuming a large haul of deep-sea mullet, the Anbarra man Michael Aningarra succinctly explained the difference between living at the government settlement, Maningrida, and at the mouth of An-gatja Wana (Blyth River). At Maningrida, he said, when a fish was purchased from the Progress Association Store, there were ten people to eat it. At Lalarr-gadjirripa, one person could have ten fish.

This story exemplifies the appreciation the Anbarra have for their wholesome and plentiful diet, and emphasizes their good fortune. It also introduces an opposition — that between Maningrida and Lalarr-gadjirripa, between European town life and that in the bush — which forms the basis of many contemporary Aboriginal concepts about physical and mental well-being.

A common assumption made by health professionals and others is that Aborigines do not appreciate the benefits of nutritious food and therefore need to be told what constitutes a balanced diet and how such food should be cooked. Not only are those views ethnocentric and patronizing, they are also inaccurate. It is true of Aborigines as it is of the bulk of the European population in Australia, that they do not possess a detailed understanding of the basis of human nutrition. However, their approach to the selection of food, its preparation and cooking indicates that they do have well-defined ideas about what constitutes a balanced diet. It is when these same people find themselves in alien situations that their solution to dietary imperatives breaks down. On mission-stations, government settlements and on the fringes of towns, Aborigines cannot continue to put their knowledge into practice. Here, where their wages are low and they no longer have access to bush foods, they resort to flour, tea and sugar. To know what constitutes a nutritious diet is of no use whatsoever if you are unable to procure the components of that diet.

The Anbarra, Gidjingali-speaking Aborigines, own about 50

square kilometres of extraordinarily resource-rich land, which is draped around the mouth of the Blyth River. They also have defined foraging rights over an equally productive 180 square kilometres adjacent to their land, which is owned by neighbouring groups with whom they have close social ties. In 1957, the government outpost at Maningrida was set up about 40 kilometres to the west of An-gatja Wana, on Gunavidji land. Many Anbarra people moved there immediately, as did representatives of the Gunbalang, Gungoragoni, Gunwing-gu, Gunavidji, Gunadba, Nakara, Djinang and Yanyango.

The people who settled at Maningrida in the late 1950s not only moved on to alien soil to live with many potentially hostile people, but by so doing, also gave up the economic basis of what had been their existence up to that time — the wide variety of animal and plant foods that their estates provided and on which they and their ancestors had lived for thousands of years. Some people began to forage for food in areas adjacent to Maningrida, but because these resources did not belong to them, and because so many people were predating upon a tract of land that previously had provided for a much smaller group, food supplies soon dwindled.

The situation started to change in about 1970, as the tensions and deprivations of town life began to have their effect on the population (Meehan and Jones, 1980). Many people, including some Anbarra, returned to their own territories, where they established what have become known as outstations. There they resumed a life largely pre-European in structure but incorporating elements of European culture, by then considered necessary features of the neo-hunting lifestyle.

The people who left Maningrida after fifteen years were articulate about the wisdom of their decision and the superiority of their life in the bush. They were pleased to be once more curating their own territory, cleaning the waterholes and burning the land, as they had done so productively in the past, and to be camping close to their totemic sites, because these play a vital role in their lives. With land rights so much in the news at the time, the Aborigines also felt that they were sensible to be sitting on their own land, "holding it tight", until the government took steps to make sure that, in terms of European law, it belonged to them forever. This in fact became a reality only in 1976, with the passage of the *Land Rights Act (Northern Territory)* 1976 through federal parliament, which gave freehold title of reserve land to Aboriginal owners.

Aborigines also were relieved to be away from Maningrida, where they had to listen to so many languages and where they had been constantly exposed to dangerous acts performed by sorcerers. Illnesses and deaths that occurred in the town often were attributed

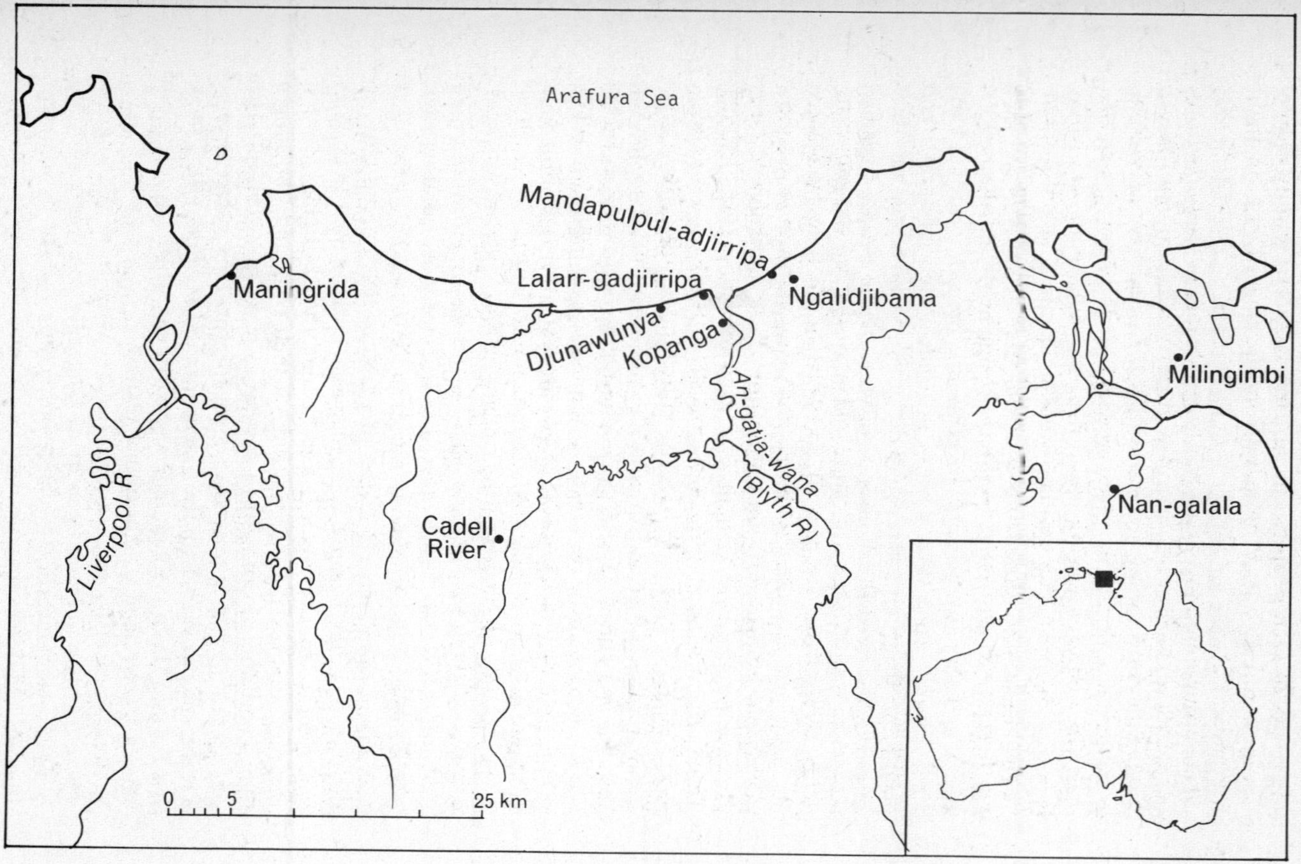

Map 3. North-central Arnhem Land

to the work of such people. The Anbarra felt that the only escape from these threats was to be away from the town, living on their own land.

The most commonly cited advantage of being on the outstations was that there, bush food was once more available in abundance. The diet the Anbarra enjoyed during 1972–73, and have continued to savour since that time, gives credence to this view, especially when it is compared with the food that the same people ate while they were living at Maningrida: bread or damper (an unleavened bread made from flour and water), tinned meat and breakfast cereal, and perhaps the occasional helping of fresh meat or fish.

RESOURCES

Anbarra land is ecologically varied and thus rich in food and technological resources (Meehan, 1975 : 19–21, 40–72; Jones, 1980). Its mosaic of open woodlands, black soil plains, freshwater swamps and lagoons, old inland dunes, monsoon thickets, mangroves and vast stretches of open beach and sea, each provide a suite of foods that are exploited during the annual cycle according to a complex set of limiting factors such as seasonality and weather conditions.

The information about Anbarra diet presented here is based on data collected during several periods of fieldwork in the Liverpool and Blyth River areas: two years at Maningrida in 1958 and 1960, and one month in 1970; and a series of field trips in 1972, 1973, 1974 and 1978, totalling about twenty months, during which time a detailed study of the diet of the Anbarra people and the resources available on their territory was made.[1]

Shellfish and Crustacea

Anbarra eat about thirty species of shellfish, the most important being the gastropod *Melo amphora* and the bivalves *Batissa violacea*, *Modiolus micropterus*, *Anadara granosa*, *Mactra meretriciformis* and *Tapes hiantina*. The latter, highly prized *diyama*, contributed 67 per cent of the total gross weight of shellfish eaten during 1972–73.

Some six species of fresh and saltwater crustacea are included in the diet. The most important is the large mud crab *Scylla serrata*, found in the intertidal zone and mangrove forest. At certain times, prawns (e.g. *Parapenaeopsis sculptilis*) are captured from the same areas with nets made from plant fibres.

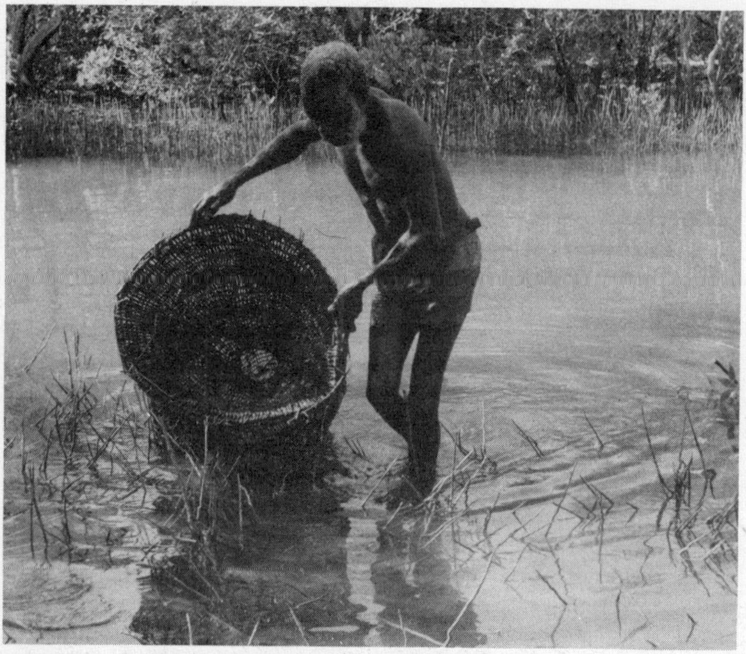

Gurrmanamana removing a fish-trap from the tidal creek at Gunadjangga, a site lying a few kilometres to the west of Lalarr-gadjirripa.

Fish

Fish, including stingrays and sharks, are regularly eaten, approximately sixty different species being procured from freshwater billabongs and creeks, tidal creeks and the intertidal zone, using a range of fishing techniques such as the three-pronged fish spear and spear-thrower, fish-traps, nets and, nowadays, European nylon fishing-lines and metal hooks. Species that contribute most include the ubiquitous barramundi *Lates calcarifer*, six species of cat-fish, of which *Hexanematichthys leptaspis* is most commonly caught, the highly prized deep-sea mullet *Lisa dussumieri* and several species of stingray, including the large *Dasyatis* cf. *lubricus.*

Reptiles

This important category of turtles, lizards and snakes includes fresh- and salt-water species, those providing most to the diet being goannas (*Varanus* spp), freshwater turtles (three genera) and

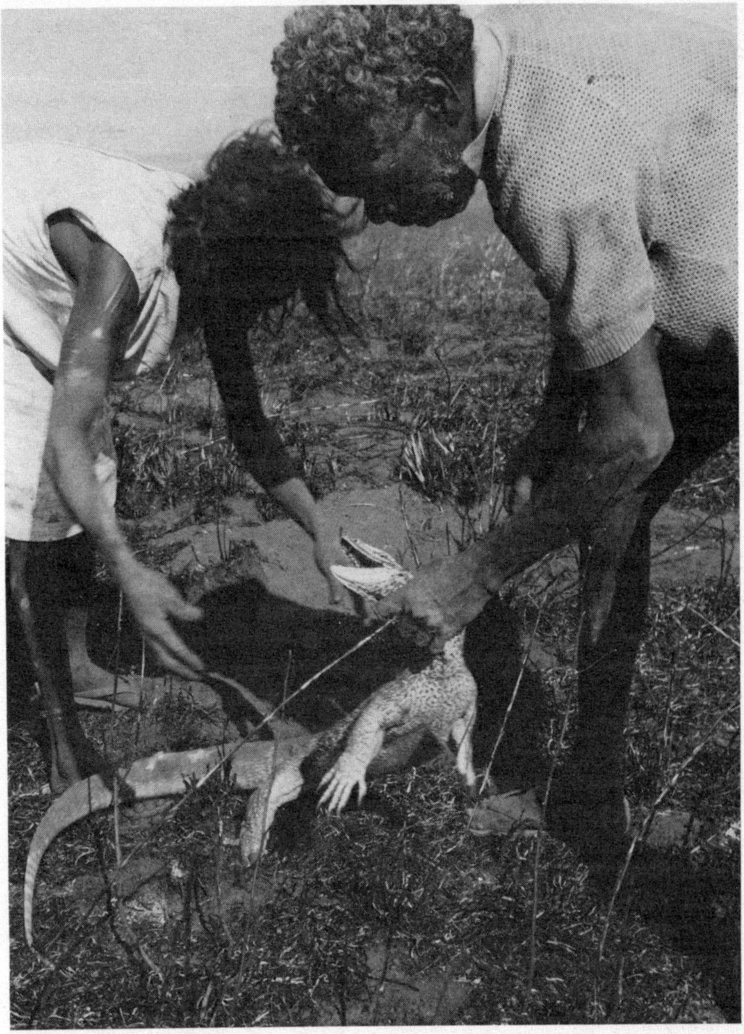

Bandeiyama (*left*) and Gurrmanamana maiming a goanna that they have just dug from the hole behind them.

pythons. Occasionally large salt-water turtles are harpooned, but the smaller reptiles contribute more consistently to the daily fare. Reptilian eggs are sought eagerly during the rainy period of the year. Large hauls of up to a hundred salt-water turtle eggs frequently are brought into the camp.

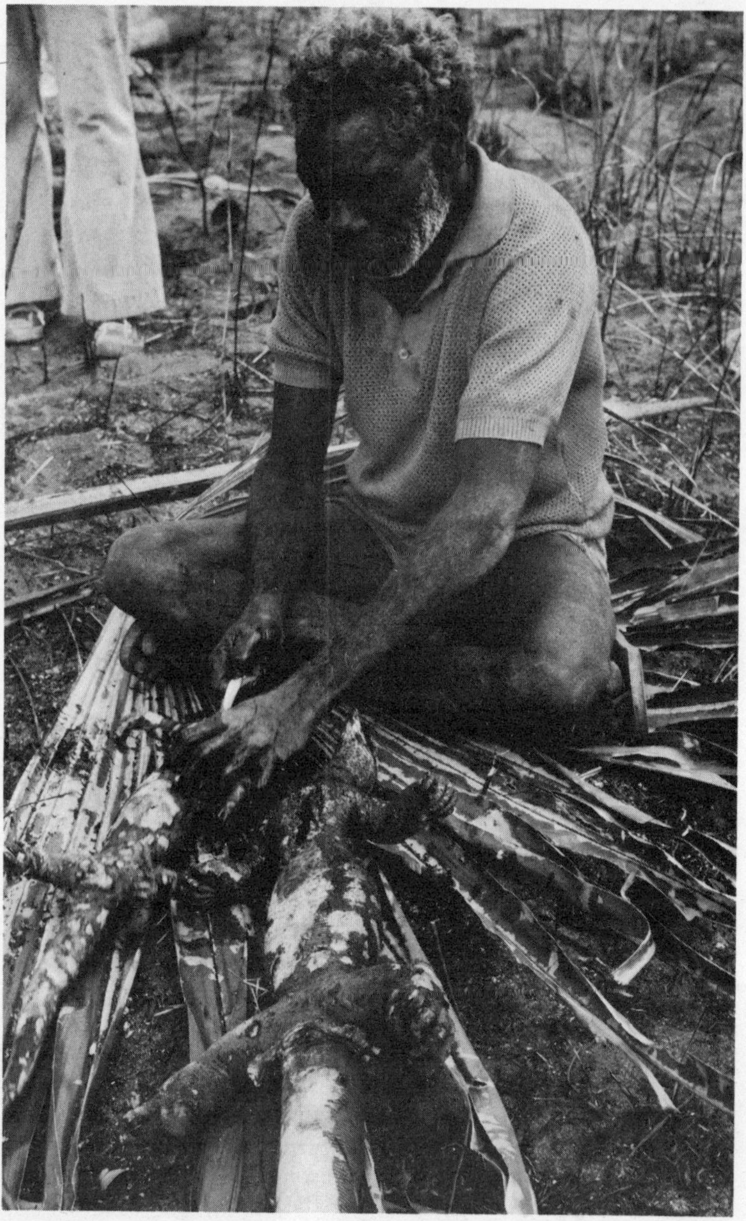

A later stage in the butchering of a goanna. Gurrmanamana is sitting on a *gangila* (*Corypha* sp.) palm.

Birds

Coastal Arnhem Land abounds with bird life, and the Anbarra stalk many species and gather their eggs. It is likely, due to the fact that some Aboriginal hunters possess .22 rifles and shot-guns, that a wider range of birds is procured now than prior to the introduction of European weapons. However, species that form a significant part of contemporary diet — for example, the large black and white magpie goose *Anseranas semipalmata* — also were important in the past. Their accessibility is related to the behaviour of the birds, the fact that they congregate in vast numbers at predictable times of the year (Gaughwin, 1978 : 1–14), rather than to the way in which they are caught. Any adequate technology deployed at optimum times ensures a good yield. In the past, Anbarra goose-harvesting strategies involved a large group of men armed with bundles of goose spears and a spear-thrower. They stalked the birds in freshwater swamps, as they do today with guns, and as the geese rose to escape the intruders, hurled their spears in rapid succession into the cloud of feathers, killing and wounding many animals. After a short time, the surviving geese resettled on the swamp to feed, and the hunters repeated their attack. Frank Gurrmanamana, an Anbarra man of great knowledge and experience, insists that using this technique, men were able to capture as many geese as they do today with shot-guns, though it may have taken them longer to do so. Other important species that appear on the menu are ducks (e.g. *Anas superciliosa*), brolgas *Grus rubicunda*, ibis *Threskiornis molucca* and jabiru *Xenorhynchus asiaticus.* The large and unwise plains turkey *Eupodotis australis* falls easy prey to Anbarra hunters, and its flesh is considered to be excellent red meat.

Mammals

Only a few mammals — wallabies, kangaroos, feral cats and some small marsupial mice and rats — inhabit Anbarra territories, and they are less important in the diet in terms of total weight than other resources. Wallabies, *Macropus agilis*, are the most commonly eaten. They are especially important on the western bank of An-gatja Wana, where they abound. On the eastern bank, where the Anbarra own only a limited area of land, the larger kangaroo *M. antilopinus* takes their place. Increasingly the exotic buffalo *Bubalus bubalis*, introduced last century from South-east Asia, roams the black-soil plains of the north and drinks from the swamps. As the Anbarra are only just beginning to perfect a strategy for hunting these creatures, they appear infrequently in the diet. This red meat is highly prized.

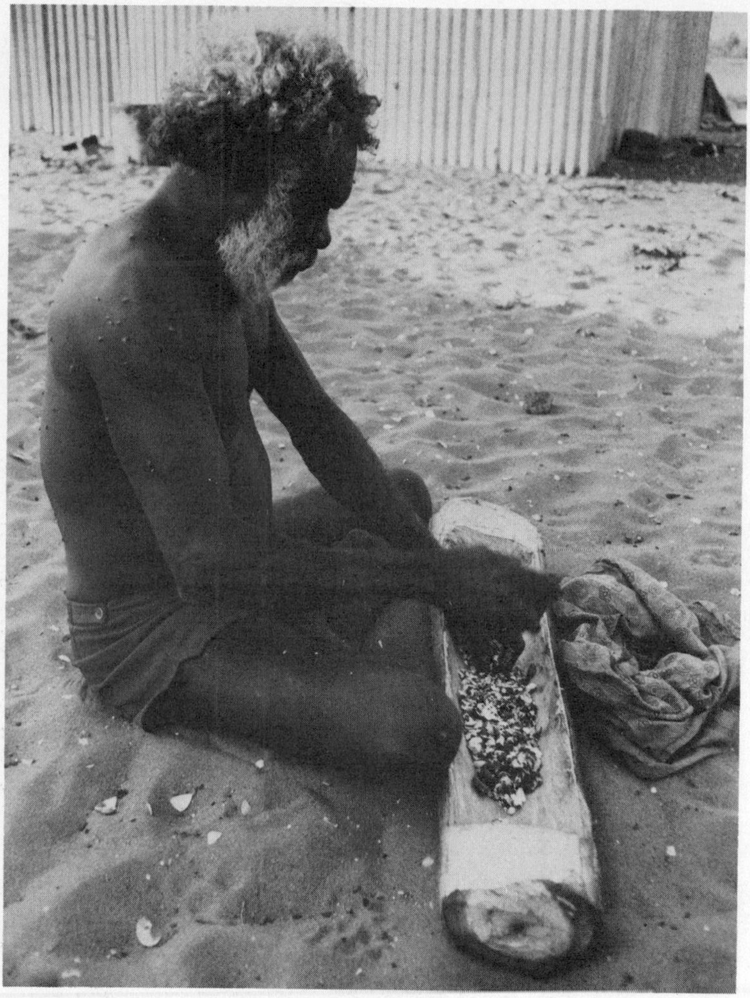

Gurrmanamana crushing the corms from the spike rush *Eleocharis dulcis* at the Anbarra home-base Kopanga. The wooden bowl is a traditional utensil. The corm is crushed with a river pebble.

Plant Foods

The Anbarra are fortunate to have a wide range of plant foods available on their territory. The most important tuber, *Dioscorea transversa*, is available during the early to middle part of the dry season and is retrieved from the many monsoon thickets in the area.

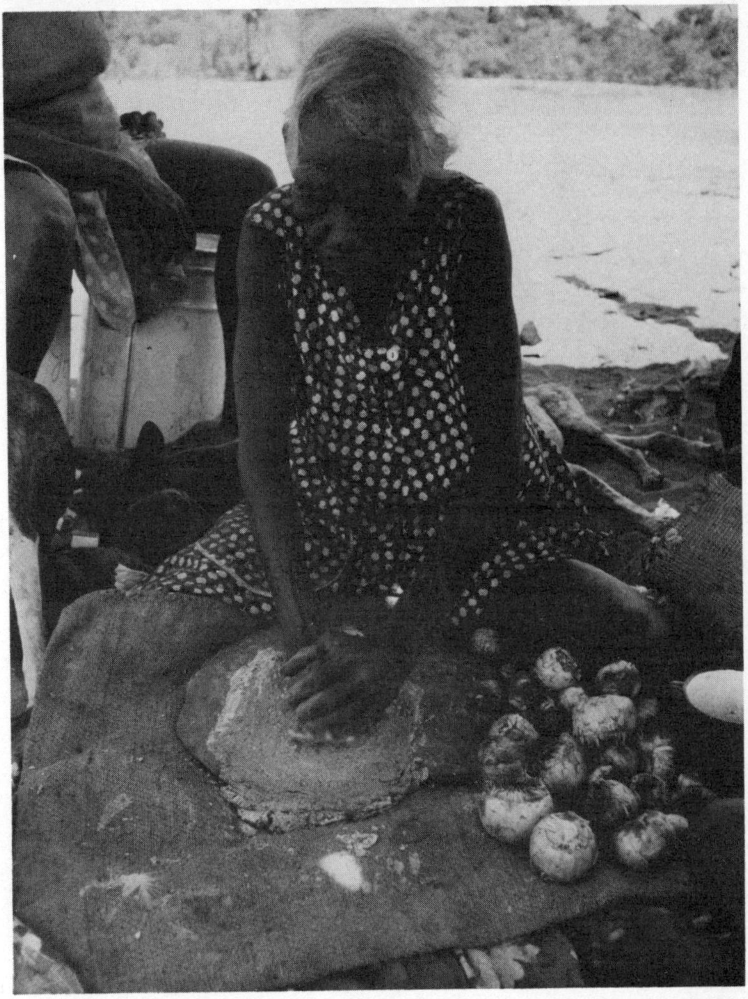

Marrkoweitj preparing some unleavened bread from the seeds of the water lily (*Nymphaea* sp.) at Djunawunya home-base. Unground seeds are seen on right.

The corm of the spike rush *Eleocharis dulcis*, known as *kuleitj*, is gathered by women while men are catching geese. The latter congregate on freshwater swamps specifically to eat this plant. The same swamps contain a wide range of edible products, which are processed from several species of water plants, especially water lilies

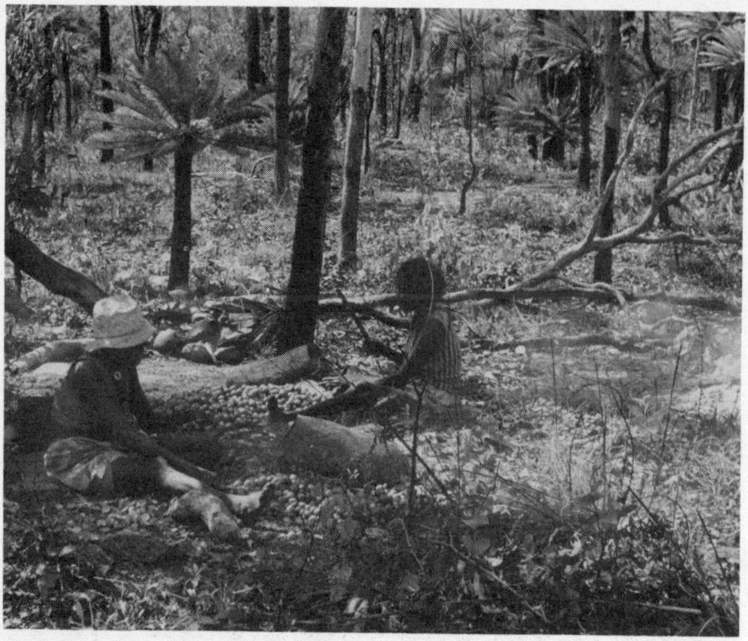

Women preparing *Cycas media* in forest on the eastern side of An-gatja Wana, near the home-base Ngalidjibama. The palms in the background are Cycad trees. The flesh from the Cycad ovule is crushed, then soaked in water for about five days. This removes the toxin. Finally the crushed flesh is made into loaves, which are baked in an earth oven.

Nymphaea sp. From the woodlands, where the eucalypts *Eucalyptus tetradonta* flourish, the ovules of the highly toxic plant *Cycas media* are gathered. This plant forms a major part of the diet during the early dry season, when important ceremonies are performed and for which reliable and abundant supplies of staple foods are required. This food is subjected to a complex process of drying, leaching and baking, designed to remove the toxin Cycasin, before it is eaten as bread (Beaton, 1977 : 160–81; Meehan and Jones, 1977).

Fruits of many sizes and tastes burst in and out of season throughout the year; their arrivals and departures are discussed by gatherers with knowledge and expectation. The most popular of the fruits are the "red apple" *Syzigium suborbiculare* and *Morinda citrifolia*, both of which are ready to eat about Christmas-time; the large, pale-green fruit of the latter lasts throughout the wet, sometimes well into the early dry season. The delicious kernels of *Pandanus* (probably *P. spiralis*) are ready to harvest by the middle of the year, between July and October, and their small, oily, energy-packed kernels are a great favourite (Meehan, Gaffey and Jones, 1979). In the early dry season, fruits from several trees, such as the spherical, dark-red berries from *Mimusops elengi* and the small, green, furry fruit produced by *Terminalia carpentariae*, become avail able.

Miscellaneous Food

This abundant repertoire of major foods is enhanced by the addition of a variety of small foods that are valued by the Anbarra people, such as the larvae of beetles and moths (witchetty-grubs), honey from the hives of wild bees and termites that are collected from several types of nests.

European Food

The Anbarra supplement their diet these days with European foods. They favour white flour and white sugar, but also buy smaller quantities of white rice and porridge. Children purchase soft drinks when they are available and the adults, mainly men, are fond of alcohol. Some Anbarra people say that one of the reasons they left Maningrida was to get away from "too many drunken men", and it is noticeable that on the outstations, people drink less alcohol and alcohol-induced conflicts are rare. Some outstations have banned alcohol altogether. Aboriginal consumption of alcohol, on outstations as well as in towns, is a continuing target for derogatory press comment. While there is no doubt that excessive alcohol consumption is a problem for some Aboriginal communities, it does appear that in some cases comment has been ill-informed (Meehan and Jones, 1980).

To a certain extent, European carbohydrate foods have replaced indigenous plant foods, though the most popular of the latter still form part of the diet when they are in season. In some ways, they are more valued now than they were in the past, because they are collected in smaller quantities much less frequently. Based on discussions held with knowledgeable Anbarra people, it has been argued (Meehan, 1975 : Appendix 6) that the structure of their contemporary diet is much the same as it was in the past, even though some of the specific items in it have changed. People still eat approximately the same amount of meat and plant food as they did before the arrival of the Europeans, the difference being that now the latter includes flour and sugar, as well as the best of the bush vegetables.

NOTHING BUT THE BEST

The Anbarra, living on their own land, are an unusually food-conscious group of people. They seek and acquire ingredients of the highest quality and prepare, cook and present them with imagination and care. Because they live in an area so rich in food, they are able to pick and choose from their abundant larder. They also discriminate within categories, and take the best in terms of their own needs, tastes and desires. For example, they do not eat crocodile, nor do they eat every species of snake. "Poison" snakes are never gathered, but other snakes, including pythons and a small non-venomous species called *manmarrkmanmarrk*, are considered to be delicacies. Some shellfish, which are freely available throughout the year, *Telescopium telescopium* and *Terebralia palustris*, are collected rarely, despite the fact that they are edible and occur in large numbers in accessible places. The same people who reject these gastropods will walk several kilometres to gather, from a mangrove area where there is no fresh water and a host of mosquitoes, the large chunky bivalve *Batissa violacea*, which has a low flesh to shell ratio (12 per cent). They say that they like its "salty taste". These few examples demonstrate that the Anbarra are not, as Aborigines sometimes popularly have been portrayed, a people living from day to day, eking out an existence by eating every edible product available to them.

The rules for acceptance appear to be similar for most items, though of course the details of the standards vary with the particular product and the gathering situation. People prefer "young" plants and animals to those that are "old"; they also savour "fat" characteristics, not "thin" ones, and all display definite preference for "fresh" food as opposed to that that has been procured a day, sometimes even only a few hours, before. They do not like food, especially fruits and nuts, that is "not ready", preferring that that is ripe and tasty. The most complimentary thing a person can say about any food is that it is *molamola* ("good" or "sweet").

In the case of shellfish, people specifically seek "big" and "fat" specimens. Small individuals are discarded. The great mud crab comes under close scrutiny from collectors. Those that are thin are discarded. Unlike Europeans, the Anbarra prefer body flesh to that in the legs and claws. The fish species most favoured by the Anbarra are cat-fish and deep-sea mullet. They dislike "big" or "old" specimens, preferring those about 20 cm long; they relish fish that comes directly from the water and is placed on the coals of the cooking fire. When stingrays and sharks are captured, they are butchered always, so that their livers can be inspected. If these are not up to standard, the animals are discarded. When Frank Gurrmanamana, a senior Anbarra man, was on a visit to the author in Canberra, a special purchase of snapper was made for dinner, since it was known how much he liked fish and how he missed not having it regularly when he came south. Frank was most suspicious when the fish was taken from the freezer. He held it up close to his eyes, inspecting every detail, saying: "Old one, aye?" During the wet season at Lalarr-gadjirripa, a young man, Sam Gumugun, caught a groper (probably *Promicrops lanceolatus*) weighing more than 140 kg with a 12 kg fishing-line. Everyone was excited about the catch and it was obvious that Sam was greatly respected for his prowess. However, after the great mound of flesh had been dragged up above the high-tide mark, Gumugun's father cut one 2 kg steak from its tail, more as a gesture towards his son than because he wanted the flesh. The rest was left on the beach to rot.

Birds are thrown away rarely. This is probably because they form only a small and highly seasonal part of the diet and consequently are valued for the novelty of their flavour rather than for the quality of their flesh. In any case, most birds, especially those living in water environments, are captured when they are in good condition, when they are feeding on water plants. Even so, hunters choose especially fat geese for themselves before they distribute the balance of their catch. All mammals are classified as "red meat" and form a valued part of the diet. Only once have macropod carcasses been observed left uneaten.

Although people are vocal about the quality of various plant foods they eat, they appear to be less discerning with these than with flesh foods. Perhaps this is due, as with birds, to the highly seasonal nature of most plants and the fact that the Anbarra generally collect them at optimum times.

Before the introduction of tea and other beverages, the main liquid available to Aborigines was water. Sometimes they mix with this wild honey and the sweet pith from the trunk of the palm *Livistona humilis* and *Carpentaria acuminata*. Everyone is meticulous about cleaning waterholes, about removing debris from within and around these sources. The Anbarra have clear ideas about what constitutes "good water", though at times they are forced to drink from wells that they do not like. Water from the large, deep wells situated beneath the deep shade of the fig trees at the coastal site Mandapulpul-adjirripa, on the eastern bank of the Blyth River, is considered to be the best water in the area; it is clear and "all the same ice water".

Most Anbarra today are familiar with European food. They buy large quantities of flour, sugar and rice. They favour "white" rather than "brown" products. The Anbarra also buy small quantities of salt, which traditionally was not used. They are interested in soup and stews, knowledge of the latter being acquired by the older men and women when they were members of buffalo and timber camps in their youth. In general, they do not like tinned meat, and if forced to eat it, always remove the cold, tasteless layer of fat that invariably surrounds it.

RAW AND COOKED

There is a widespread misconception that Aborigines are indifferent cooks: that they throw a carcass on to a fire, cook it for a few minutes, then pull it apart with great haste, as if they have not eaten for six months. This is certainly not true of the Anbarra. Most food is cooked. Traditional techniques include the use of dry and moist ovens, grilling and some forms of stewing.

The "mangrove worm" is always eaten raw. This highly valued animal is collected from rotting logs in mangrove forests. Mud is squeezed from its alimentary canal before the soft body is eaten.

Most shellfish are cooked before they are eaten, except in situations where people are collecting oysters, mussels or *Tapes hiantina* and wish to taste one or two, to see if they are fat or how much "sweet milk" they contain.[2] As far as is known, gastropods always are cooked. Sometimes grubs are eaten raw; they also may be roasted.

Most fruit and nuts are devoured immediately they are harvested. The fruit *Mimusops elengi*, called *bulba*, a small spherical red-black berry, is eaten raw, but sometimes also is cooked in a dry oven, as are the tasty corms of the spike rush *Eleocharis dulcis*. Some plant foods that are eaten raw are prepared beforehand; for example, the crisp, "red apple" *Syzigium suborbiculare* is de-seeded, then made into a fresh and slightly astringent-tasting pulp by being placed in a long wooden mortar and pounded with a river pebble. *Eleocharis dulcis* occasionally is prepared this way, particularly if the corms are those of the mature variety and have been stored in the camp for a few days.

When the Anbarra choose to cook food, they use one of the following techniques:

Grilling

Grilling is common in all Anbarra camps, the food being placed on top of glowing coals. Here it is turned and tended until ready. Some shellfish are prepared this way. When the shells begin to sizzle and pop, they are considered ready to eat.

The most effective use of grilling is applied to the cooking of crabs and birds, though wallabies and kangaroos are prepared in a similar fashion. Live crabs are placed on the coals of a fire; sometimes the claws and legs are removed and cooked separately. This method produces crab meat that possesses a succulent flavour and is still moist with natural juices.

Geese that have been grilled on coals are tasty, and hunting men have been seen to eat one or even two birds about 1.5 kg in weight in one sitting. The butchering of geese and other birds is a complex procedure, but when the bird comes off the coals it has acquired a crisp brown skin and exudes a delicious aroma. Inside, the flesh is pink and tender. As the flesh is consumed, the larger bones are cracked to obtain the marrow.

Another dramatic grilling technique is used to cook bivalve shellfish, especially *Tapes hiantina*, *Modiolus micropterus* or *Batissa violacea*. After the shells have been washed, they are arranged with their lips pressed into a clean area of soil. A small, fast fire is then ignited on their hinges, which are set uppermost, beginning at one end. As a group of shells cook, and this can be recognized by the sounds of hissing and popping, a stick is used to move the fire along the phalanx of hinges, until all the shellfish are ready. Ashes and coals are then brushed from the scorched hinges and the aromatic-smelling shellfish are knocked from their cooking positions on to a pile of grass, where they are allowed to cool before being eaten. Shellfish cooked in this way possess a slight but pleasant smoky flavour and are always moist.

Today the Anbarra have expanded their grilling techniques by using pieces of wire mesh to cook food, in much the same way that we barbecue steak and sausages.

Stewing

A type of stewing was used by the Anbarra in the past, but it did not involve the use of water. Nowadays, liver is cooked slowly until it forms a kind of sauce. Stingray liver and fat is placed in an empty *Melo amphora* shell. This is put on a fire and left until the liver and fat have melted into what the Anbarra translate as "gravy" or "soup soup". In the meantime, the rest of the animal is prepared in a dry oven (see below). When this is completed, the flesh that has been removed from the skeleton is rinsed several times in fresh water, after which it is squeezed dry to form a fibrous mass. It is this substance, portions being picked up with the tips of the fingers, that is dipped into the gravy before being eaten.

Traditional stewing is associated with the use of a dry oven and is an integral part of cooking a large barramundi. Normally these are cooked in dry ovens, but on one occasion, at the conclusion of a communal barramundi fishing day during which about 80 kg were procured, Gurrmanamana removed the head of one fish, then cut a bowl-shaped section from the body, its ventral side forming the base. This was placed on top of a heap of glowing coals. It was supported in this position by other large coals, more of which were placed on the rim of the "bowl". The fat from the fish and its liver were placed in the cavity and for the next forty-five minutes Gurrmanamana sat patiently overseeing the process, reorganizing the fire, replacing hot coals for cold and generally giving the matter his undivided attention. When the fish was cooked, it was crisp and golden brown — like a Sunday roast — and the fish-flesh joint had formed itself into a perfect bowl. Inside, steaming and producing a delicious aroma, was about 5 cm of fatty juice. The roasted fish piece was removed from the fire and placed on a thick bed of fresh green grass; everyone sat around it, anticipating the feast. A piece of flesh broken from the bowl walls was dipped into the "soup soup" and eaten. Frank Gurrmanamana commented, with pride, that when barramundi was eaten this way, one did not need any blankets: it made one so fat and shiny that one did not feel the cold.

Roasting and the Use of Ovens

Two methods of roasting are used by the Anbarra — the dry oven and the steam oven — although there are several variations of each.

The dry oven is constructed by making a fire on a specific area, preferably of clean sand. This is allowed to die down until it is a mixture of glowing coals, hot ash and hot sand. The fire is then moved a little to one side and a depression made in the sand with a cooking-stick, which is a piece of hardwood about 1 m long and 4 cm wide. Then ashes and coals are placed on the bottom of the "oven" and covered with more hot sand, ashes and coals. Depending on the size of the object to be cooked, a small fire may be rekindled on top of the oven and/or the food may be turned halfway through cooking. The reason this cooking method is likened to that of an oven is that everything is cooked in its own container — skin or carapace — its own Dutch oven. When the food is cooked, the containers are removed and discarded. All that has been cooked is eaten. Most fish is prepared by this method, as are goannas, turtles, snakes, lizards, small rats and mice.

Many plant foods also are prepared using this type of oven; the important yam *Dioscorea transversa* responds especially well. The tubers are cooked for about thirty minutes, as described above.

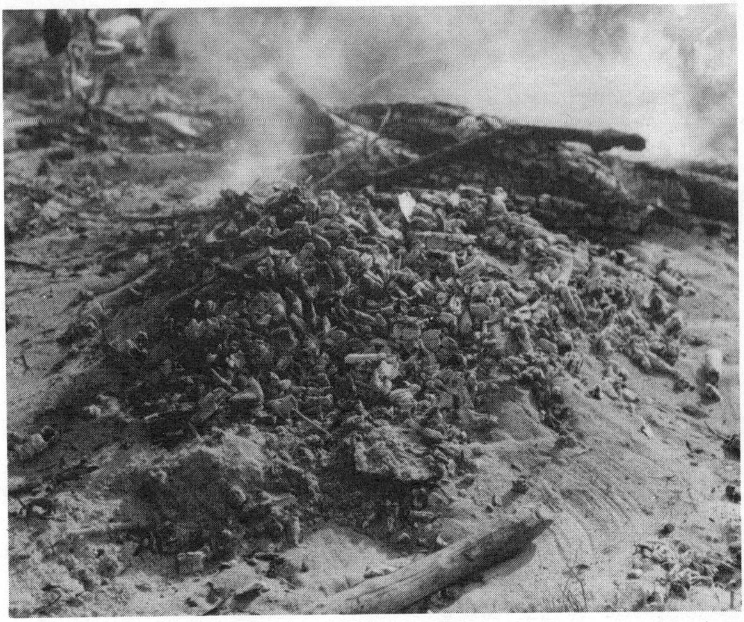

A dry oven in use.

They then are removed from the oven and are dusted with a fresh green branch and placed on a pile of grass to cool before they are eaten. Dampers made with flour and water, and more recently with flour, baking powder and sometimes even dried fruits, also are prepared in dry ovens.

The steam oven is an impressive piece of cooking technology. There are two models. The one used on the coast utilizes dead shells and is constructed only to cook shellfish; in inland areas, shells are replaced with pieces of ant-bed and the ovens are used to cook kangaroo, emu and buffalo. A large fire is kindled and allowed to burn down to a bed of glowing coals. Considerable quantities of dead shells or pieces of ant-bed about 12 cm in diameter are thrown on the coals and mixed with them. If shellfish are being cooked, they are tipped on the heated dead shells, green branches are placed over them and the oven is sealed with paperbark. Everybody sits around the oven, holding down the paperbark, to ensure that no steam escapes. In two or three minutes, the cooking is done. If a buffalo is to be prepared, the bones are removed where possible and the meat is cut into large joints. These are mixed with the heated ant-bed nodules. The meat is placed on the coals and the entire construction is then covered with a thick layer of green branches, bark and, if possible, earth. If the preparation begins in the late afternoon, the meat is left to cook overnight.

Some European cooking methods have been adopted by the Anbarra, together with some European food. The most important of these is boiling. Butchered wallaby, fish, crab and shellfish are boiled in drums of salt water or fresh water to which salt has been added. At the moment, boiling constitutes only a small portion of cooking (say 5 per cent). When it is used, it invariably means a deterioration of cooking standards and consequent loss of much of the nutritive value of many foods. People also prepare porridge, rice and several flour dishes in billy-cans and saucepans.

One of the features of Anbarra life that is constantly impressive is the simple but attractive way in which the people present their food. Products always are cleaned carefully before they are cooked, and all ash, coal and sand are removed by light brushing with a small branch of fresh green leaves or by shaking the food in a dilly-bag. The food is then arranged on a thick pile of fresh green grass or leaves, or on newly gathered paperbark. People eat their meals from these platters, wiping their hands on them when they have finished.

A BALANCED DIET

For the Anbarra, all edible substances — animal and vegetable — are *gala* (flesh). Reference to specific types of flesh is qualified by one of four prefixes, depending upon the noun class to which it has been assigned (Meehan, 1975 : 85–102). Thus flesh from the shellfish *Tapes hiantina* is *an-gala* (male class), that belonging to the magpie goose is *djin-gala* (female class), that from the *Eleocharis dulcis* corm is *man-gala* (vegetable class). The flesh from the mangrove-worm is *gun-gala* (mostly inorganic class). All edible plant food is subsumed under the term *balidja*. Most European foods, especially flour and sugar are included in this category. Animal flesh is divided into:

mindjak — flesh of land and sea mammals, birds and reptiles;
djidjidjda — flesh of edible fish, including sharks and rays;
kapara — the flesh of bivalves found in open sea-shell beds;
ngal — a category that includes flesh of crustacea, insects and some shellfish, including those from mangroves.

Cutting across this division of animal flesh is the concept of "white" or "clean" flesh, exemplified by fish, shellfish and goanna, and "red" flesh or "flesh with blood inside", such as that derived from wallabies and buffaloes. Though the Anbarra eat both red and white meat, they strongly favour the latter.

The Anbarra prefer a diet that contains ample quantities of all the different food categories. If forced to eat white meat for too many days, they complain, saying they are tired of *djidjidja* (fish) and want red meat. If they have lots of flour, yams or spike rush, *balidja*, they say how much they wish to have "beef", meaning any kind of white or red animal flesh. Sometimes they crave for *balidja*, especially during the wet season when traditional and European forms are in short supply and they eat fish and crabs constantly. On a more subtle level, people sometimes say they want to have shellfish because its flesh is "wet" (i.e. moist); they are tired of eating flesh that is "dry" (i.e. usually fish and vegetable substance).

A SATISFYING MEAL

The most important meal for the Anbarra is eaten in the middle of the day. For those engaged in a hunting expedition, this invariably means that it is eaten away from home-base. Serious foraging expeditions leave home-base about ten in the morning and foraging continues until about noon. If the morning's work has been productive, a "dinner-time camp" is established where the foragers cook the food that has been procured, eat a substantial amount of it, then rest for an hour or so before commencing the afternoon's activities. If the group contains only men, this midday meal normally consists entirely of animal flesh, though they may eat small quantities of ripe fruit during their journey. Large amounts of meat are taken per head. For a foraging group of women and children, the midday meal is usually more eclectic and consists of meat and plant foods (Meehan, Gaffey and Jones, 1979). Groups of mature female hunters usually procure animal flesh as well as plant foods. On specialized trips, one variety of food constitutes the bulk of what is procured on that day.

Those who choose to stay in the camp during the day are given the food left over from "dinner-time" and a share of food that has been accumulated on the homeward journey. Evening meal also consists of what is left from midday and food acquired on the way home. For breakfast, people eat what is left from both meals, plus perhaps breakfast cereal or damper. Very sweet tea, amply supplemented with dried milk, is consumed in large quantities with every meal.

AN AMPLE FARE

There is no doubt that the Anbarra diet is varied and of high quality. Traditional cooking techniques enhance the flavour of each item and ensure a maximum retention of nutrients. Food is presented in an attractive manner and the people eat it in a relaxed environment. However, these factors can be of no consequence if the amount of food the people receive is insufficient for good health.

Data recorded during 1972–73 are discussed elsewhere (Meehan, 1975 : 103–31, 198–230; 1977a, 1977b, 1977c). The gross weight of food consumed by the Anbarra (Table 4) varied. During January (Table 5), each person received an average of 1.8 kg gross weight of food per day, equivalent to 1620 kcal; in April, it was 2.2 kg or 2400 kcal; in May, 1.8 kg or 2500 kcal; while in September 1972, it was 1.9 kg or 2090 kcal. In all months except January, Anbarra people were receiving, on average, more than a recommended intake of 2050 kcal (Meehan, 1977a : 517–18).[3] During that month, monsoon rains burst upon the small camp at Lalarr-gadjirripa. People did little else but sit, sleep and talk inside their wet-season long-houses. Few appeared to be particularly hungry and only rarely did anyone leave the security and comfort of these dwellings to collect food. Because of this inactivity, the people did not require much energy and they certainly did not complain about being hungry — only about the wind, the rain and the mosquitoes!

During 1972–73, a combination of vegetables and purchased carbohydrate food contributed 31.4 per cent (Table 6) of the gross weight of all food eaten; this was equivalent to 56.9 per cent of all the energy available to the community. It is likely that in the past, indigenous vegetables alone would have made a similar contribution to the total diet, i.e. about 50 per cent of required energy. It is clear that flour and sugar contribute substantially to the "vegetable" component of the modern diet (Table 7), i.e. 62.6 per cent of the gross weight or 89.1 per cent of the energy. During April, a month when traditional vegetable food is abundant, bush vegetables provided 46.5 per cent of the gross weight of all vegetables or only 14.5 per cent of energy. (Indigenous plants tend to contain fewer calories per unit weight than refined European products such as flour and sugar.) In the past, women would have had to work longer collecting vegetables than they do today, if these were to have provided half the energy requirement of the community (Meehan, 1975 : Appendix 6).

There is no doubt that the diet enjoyed by the Anbarra during 1972–73 was nutritious. In general, it provided an excess of a rec-

Table 4. Foods Eaten by Anbarra Community, 1972–73

	Wet		Late Wet/Early Dry		Dry		Late Dry	
	January 1973 days = 31/people = 30		April 1973 days = 30/people = 35		May 1973 days = 30/people = 37		September 1972 days = 17/people = 31	
	[a]Gross wt % 1650 kg	[b]Kcal % 1.5×10^6	Gross wt % 2280 kg	Kcal % 2.56×10^6	Gross wt % 2101 kg	Kcal % 2.88×10^6	Gross wt % 985 kg	Kcal % 1.1×10^6
Foods Hunted and Gathered								
Flesh:								
Shellfish	48.5	8.9	30.1	4.5	20.8	2.5	24.9	4.1
Crustacea	1.2	0.7	2.2	1.0	2.3	0.9	1.4	0.6
Fish	21.5	25.8	21.9	21.4	42.0	33.6	22.4	22.0
Reptiles	2.0	2.2	3.8	3.5	3.5	2.7	10.8	9.5
Birds	0.9	2.1	0.3	0.6	0.4	0.7	3.1	5.8
Mammals	5.5	13.6	0.4	0.9	—	—	8.8	17.8
Vegetables:								
Fruits and nuts	7.3	4.5	12.1	1.7	0.8	0.5	14.3	3.0
Roots/tubers	0.4	0.5	7.0	8.1	4.3	4.1	0.6	0.7
Honey	—	—	0.3	0.4	0.1	0.1	0.8	1.2
Foods Bought								
Flour and sugar	12.8	41.8	21.9	57.8	25.4	55.1	13.3	35.2

Notes:

(a) Percentage of gross weight of all food collected during January, namely 1650 kg.

(b) Percentage of amount of energy contained in all food collected during January, namely 1.5×10^6 kcal.

Table 5. Foods Eaten by Anbarra Community: Mean Intake per Head per Day, 1972–73

	Jan 1973	April 1973	May 1973	Sept 1972
Gross weight (kg)	1.8	2.2	1.8	1.9
Energy (kcal)	1620	2400	2500	2090

Table 6. Foods Eaten by Anbarra Community: Contributions Made by Vegetables and Animals, 1972–73

	All Food	Plant Food	Animal Flesh	% Contributed by Vegetables and Purchased Carbohydrate	% Contributed by Animal Flesh
Gross weight (kg)	7015.5	2200.0	4815.5	31.4	68.6
Energy (kcal)	8 040 500	4 577 000	3 463 500	56.9	43.1

Table 7. Foods Eaten by Anbarra Community: Traditional Vegetables Versus European Carbohydrate Food, 1972–73

	Jan 1973	April 1973	May 1973	Sept 1972	Total
Traditional					
Gross weight (kg)	126	435	115	147	823 (37.4%)
Energy (kcal)	76 000	252 000	131 000	41 000	500 000 (10.9%)
European					
Gross weight (kg)	212	500	534	131	1377 (62.6%)
Energy (kcal)	629 000	1 480 000	1 579 900	388 500	4 077 400 (89.1%)

ommended intake of energy and an abundant supply of protein in various forms. The diversity and freshness of foods consumed and the methods of cooking maximized trace elements and vitamins. Apart from introduced diseases, mostly now under control, the health of the Anbarra people living in the bush appears to be good. They recognize this and visiting health workers frequently comment upon it (Gillespie, Cooke & Bond, 1977 : 9).

HEALTHY MINDS

Living on their outstations, the Anbarra are fortunate: not only do they have access to European food but, more importantly, to abundant animal protein and fresh plants. This situation is, however, but one dimension of health for the Anbarra. Their emotional well-being is enhanced by the fact that they are back on their own territory after years in an alien place.

For the Anbarra, the move away from Maningrida was an intelligent act of survival; it also was an inspired example of the application of preventive medicine. In the bush, where the Anbarra are free to run their own lives as they see fit, they can think rationally about the direction in which they wish to go.

Because they now have more purpose to their lives, the Anbarra people on the outstations are healthier and happier than any of them were during the previous fifteen years at Maningrida. They have taken steps to control their own well-being, and the prognosis for their future seems substantially more optimistic than was the case under previous policies based on the paternalistic premise that other people, especially government authorities, knew what was "best for them".

NOTES

1 This study was undertaken together with a colleague, Dr Rhys Jones, Department of Prehistory, Research School of Pacific Studies, Australian National University, Canberra.

2 I have been chastised several times for eating "too many" raw oysters, being warned that I would get diarrhoea if I disobeyed. One memorable occasion on an offshore island, I disobeyed, and was duly punished (Meehan, 1975 : 157).

3 The number of kcals. in a given weight (kgm.) of food depends on the proportions of flesh, vegetable and bought foods that weight includes (Table 4); i.e. different foods contain different amounts of energy per unit weight.

REFERENCES

Allen, J., Golson, J., Jones, R., 1977. *Sunda and Sahul: Prehistoric Studies in Southeast Asia, Melanesia and Australia* (London : Academic Press).

Beaton, J., 1977. "Dangerous Harvest: Investigations in the Late Prehistoric Occupation of Upland Southeast Central Queensland" (Ph.D. thesis, Department of Prehistory, Australian National University, Canberra).

Gaughwin, D., 1978. "A Bird in the Sand: An Investigation of Muttonbirds, other Sea Birds and Waterfowl in Recent Prehistoric Southeast Australia" (B.A. (Hons) thesis, Department of Prehistory and Anthropology, Australian National University, Canberra).

Gillespie, D., Cooke, P., and Bond, D., 1977. *Maningrida Outstation Resource Centre, 1976/77 Report* (Milingimbi : Milingimbi Literature Production Centre).

Jones, R., 1980. "Hunters in the Australian Coastal Savannah" in *Human Ecology of Tropical Savannah*, ed. D. Harris and J. Weiner (London : Academic Press), pp. 107–46.

Meehan, B., 1975. "Shell Bed to Shell Midden" (Ph.D. thesis, Department of Prehistory and Anthropology, Australian National University, Canberra).

——, 1977a. "Man Does Not Live By Calories Alone: The Role of Shellfish in a Coastal Cuisine", in Allen *et al.* (1977), pp. 493–531.

——, 1977b. "Hunters by the Seashore", *Journal of Human Evolution* 6, no. 4 : 363–70.

——, 1977c. "The Role of Seafood in the Economy of a Contemporary Aboriginal Society in Coastal Arnhem Land", *Official Hansard Report*, 3 May (Canberra : Australian Government Publishing Service), pp. 1085–95.

—— and Jones, Rhys, 1977. "Preliminary Comments on the Preparation of *Cycas media* by the Gidjingali of Coastal Arnhem Land", in Beaton (1977), Appendix IV.

—— and ——, 1980. "The Outstation Movement and Hints of a White Backlash", in *Northern Australia: Options and Implications*, ed. Rhys Jones (Canberra : Research School of Pacific Studies, Australian National University), pp. 131–57.

——, Gaffey, Prue, and Jones, Rhys, 1979. "Fire to Steel: Aboriginal Exploitation of Pandanus and Some Wider Implications", in *Readings in Material Culture*, ed. P. Lauer, Occasional Papers in Anthropology 9 (St Lucia : Anthropology Museum, University of Queensland), pp. 73–96.

6
Sickness and Health in Western Arnhem Land: A Traditional Perspective

Catherine H. Berndt

> People co-operated well with treatment, but a large proportion of the community did not yet believe the facts relating to the mode of infestation by this parasite [hookworm], despite much and varied teaching. This greatly retarded the control of this disease.[1]

This statement about the Aboriginal community at Oenpelli, western Arnhem Land, added: "The general health of the community was reasonably good. Upper respiratory infections and fungal infections of the skin were the most common complaints." But the hookworm comment is especially interesting because it distinguishes between two different facets of response to health care programmes: acceptance of physical treatment at the level of procedures and techniques, and rejection of the notions of causation that go with that treatment. Even when there is agreement on diagnosis, in the sense that "the situation includes a problem", "here is something that needs attention", that agreement need not extend to the sort of problem it is, or "how it came about" – or, beyond a certain range of specifics, "what to do about it".

There are still some officials who claim that if Aboriginal people knew more about the nature and transmission of disease (for instance), they would accept the total package available to them through medical and health care services, a package that includes definitions and causation statements about prevention as well as about curing and healing. More recently, another kind of orientation is emerging in "community health" programmes. It goes beyond narrow definitions of health and sickness and tries to take into account the whole environment, physical and social. In that respect, it is moving closer to traditional Aboriginal views on the subject.

Oenpelli, now an Aboriginal community and not a mission station, is in the Arnhem Land Aboriginal Reserve. The Reserve has been Aboriginal land since 1976 when the *Land Rights Act (N.T.) 1976* was declared. Western Arnhem Land stretches from Croker and Goulburn Islands and the adjacent mainland and islands in the north, to the East Alligator River in the west, the Liverpool River in the east and the approximate headwaters of these two rivers in the south. In the late 1940s and early 1950s, conditions were very different indeed from what they are now;[2] but even then, the traditional Aboriginal cultures had been under formidable pressure for a long time. Almost all the original population of the plains and coastal islands between the East Alligator River and Darwin had died, largely from disease or violence. The Maung of the Goulburn Islands and nearby coast, their western neighbours the Yiwadja and their eastern neighbours the Walang (Gunbalang) retained their respective languages and something of their culture. Gunwinggu-speakers (including Maiali and Dangbun), moving northward and westward into and beyond the Oenpelli area, had been able to retain more of their traditional practices, not only memories of them. A few people spoke English, with varying fluency. Alcohol was not anything like the problem it became later, and mineral developments were not even a cloud on the horizon.

The Aboriginal perspective on health was not spelt out in a single formula. Different facets become prominent on different occasions, but interlinking them all was the verbal patterning that provided coherence and consistency, even in the face of apparent contradictions or discrepancies. Throughout the region, traditional Aboriginal religion was still of crucial importance, even where its active ritual expression had been reduced or halted. And a major component was myth — myth in the positive, anthropological sense.

THE DIMENSION OF MYTH

Because the Aborigines were non-literate people, depending predominantly on oral transmission, myth was a storehouse of practical information as well as of precepts. It covered all aspects of the local scene, from religious premises, ritual activities, and the nature and meaning of life, to ordinary everyday matters. The most sacred, ritual-linked myths, especially those in song form, were bound by stricter transmission rules. Others were more flexible. A story-teller could mention some issues briefly, or elaborate on details — what to do, how to do it, when, where, and perhaps why. Health or normal well-being usually were implicit in the background, unless they were threatened in some way. The routine ingredients of story-narrative were food-collecting and preparation, making and using material equipment and shelter, social relationships, gift-exchange, betrothal arrangements, taboos and avoidances, with dramatic highlights of sickness, accident, injury, jealousy, quarrelling and death. All of these concerned particular territories and sites, associated with individual persons and with named groups. These relationships sometimes were noted in the course of a story, but more often they were not, except in teaching children. Mostly they were part of the taken-for-granted information that the listeners did not need to be told about, or points that could be discussed outside the immediate story context.

Places of "Poison" or "Sickness"

Some myths refer to "dangerous" or taboo (*djamun*) places, to be avoided because of natural features (e.g. strong tide-rips), or potentially hostile spirit-associations, or because sickness or "poison" of some kind is inherent in them. One such place is Wurudja Island, near Croker Island, in Margu and Garig country. (See Berndt and Berndt, 1970 : 14, 197–98.) "Nobody goes there now, where sickness is. Only people of that country can go there, and ask, and then they don't get sick. It's all right for them to get meat and fish there, where that place made itself dangerous."

> In the pre-human era, the wife of Sickness-Dreaming Man at Wurudja bore a son. When he was old enough, they let him visit her Yiwadja relatives on the mainland with her brother, his uncle. When they were almost there, his uncle warned him, "We'd better rest in the shade for a while, because you might get too hot from this strong sun — and that would 'make us wrong', so we'd all die. We'll wait until it's cool . . ." Later, he told the others that the boy's father was Sickness-Dreaming. ("Like measles, like a very bad cold," the narrator commented.) "Don't go close to the boy, don't wake him up, don't touch his head!" All the girls secretly wanted that boy, and three made advances to him. Their husbands were jealous and killed them by sorcery, and the boy too. His uncle took the death-message home. After the first mourning, the boy's father got ready. He took hot ashes from the fire and threw them into his own eyes, blinding himself. His bones went like ashes, like concentrated sickness. His spirit, a Sickness spirit, is still there. Before he died, he called the name of the place where those people were living. Sickness rose up like a wind, blowing straight towards them, going in search of them. It was just before sunrise. The sky glowed red, like reflections from a fire. Those people thought, perhaps, that the moon and the sun were rising together. But it was that sickness coming to burn them, like hot ashes going into their bodies when they breathed, like smoke going every way from mosquito fires. And, for us, if we feel sick with that hot sickness, from wet ground, coughing and making it hard for us to breathe, we know that it comes from that place, from Wurudja, from that Sickness-Dreaming . . .

This is a mainland version, only summarized here, told early in 1950 by Mangurug, an elderly Gunwinggu woman with Maung and Yiwadja connections.[3] At Goulburn Island in 1947, Mondalmi, Lazarus Lamilami's sister, explained Wurudja from a Maung coastal-and-island perspective. The original Sickness site, she said, was at Ngarag, "Poison Point", on North Goulburn Island. Aadjag the Turtle Woman lived there. It was so dangerous that even people of that country took special precautions when visiting it. Suddenly, at the end of World War II, Aadjag went away to Wurudja, "to be with her mother – she was her mother's only daughter." That's why Wurudja is so dangerous now. Modalmi and others later expanded on the story. In a 1964 version, two young men carrying a death-message went to Wurudja to get eggs, but one of them killed a turtle there. A fiery sickness came up like a red moon, burning hot, and spread over the land, killing almost everyone. Only a little boy and girl escaped into a cave. They had to wait two months, before it was cool enough to come outside again.

Another "poison" place is near Mount Borradaile on the mainland, near Lanka (Langa). In a story from Lamilami (1974 : 26), a man named Marulda "got some *guiag*, a poison, from a place nearby that is *djang* . . . He put the poison in the ashes of a fire at the entrance of the cave, and fanned the ashes so all the smoke went into this cave. So all the people died there." The locale is a highly tabu place, with skeletal material that (at least until very recently) local Aborigines insisted was not to be touched or moved. Women, forbidden to enter the actual cave, described this poison as a "pretty red colour".

Other such places are also a source of "actual poison". Simply going near a particular place or touching a rock or breaking a rock leads automatically to disaster. (See R. M. Berndt, 1970 : 15, 18, 19, 39; the first of these mentions a Chickenpox Dreaming rock.) One mainland site near the King River was associated with choking coughs and blocked noses: "It's dangerous," women from that area warned. "We don't break sticks there, or dig for yams, or get paperbark. We might get sick, and die. We don't go near that place."

In myth, however, *any* place can be dangerous, depending on what the characters do there. If they make too much noise, or interfere with the ground by digging too hard for water, the Rainbow Snake is likely to come and swallow them in a great flood – and later vomit their bones at various sites, where their spirits still remain today as (for example) distinctive rock formations. Stories of this kind are very numerous. (See Berndt and Berndt, 1970 : 20–24; 1964 : 251–53.)

A point to remember is that even sites labelled "dangerous" are static: they cannot move about, to spread illness or trouble beyond their own boundaries. To be dangerous outside that range, they have to be activated or touched or used by *people*.

Two Stories of Sorcery-Death

This story was told by Mangurug early in 1950, at Oenpelli.

> Two Leech-Dreaming sisters came from the south-west into Gunwinggu territory. Their adventures included sweetheart relationships, but they rebuffed an old man from Gurudjmug who made eager advances to them. ("I'm starving for women!") ("You're old, and we're young!") They went on, to Gumader. He brooded about this ("listening to himself"). Then he got white clay and yellow ochre and searched among the rocks for a smooth, flat surface. He drew them there at Yirga-bimdjan, in his own country, Gurudjmug. He drew a bird too, an "eagle", "eating their hearts". He went away, "singing" that bird to kill them. The girls had been moving about, foraging for food and meat. That image, that bird, followed them and perched high on a tree above their camp. It came inside them, eating their hearts, in a dream. It seemed to them like a dream, but it was true. They lay there, weak and sick, covering themselves with sheets of paperbark. Their breathing grew fainter, and finally stopped. As they lay there, they turned into stone, at Bobongdi, a Leech place, in Gumader.

Mangurug added: "When people are sick, they pull the paperbark up to their shoulders. When they are dying, someone else pulls it right over them, and keeps a hand on that person's heart to feel when it stops beating."

The second story, told at Oenpelli early in 1950 by Nganalgindja, is very long and detailed. It is on a familiar local theme: a girl's rejection of her betrothed husband.

> Her parents scolded and beat her, but she kept running away from him. He was angry and jealous, suspecting that she preferred another man. When her parents took her part, he threatened to kill her. They yielded, but she still resisted him. One day when she was digging for yams, he sneaked up behind her, speared her in the back of the neck, and collected some of the blood in a small paperbark container. He waited for the "right colour", throwing away the blood that was "too dark". Then he heated a spear-blade to smooth over and close the wound, and called to the sorcerer-spirit, the patron of sorcerers, Nagidgid, asking him to restore her temporarily to life. Hiding behind a tree, he swung his spear-thrower to revive her. She sat up and rubbed her hand over her face: "Oh, why do we always fall into a heavy sleep after eating?" She felt weak, but she got up and stretched herself, hung her basket from her forehead, and picked up her stick. Then she saw a bird close to her. She seized it and ate it

> raw, feathers and all. Her husband, watching, said, "I've done it properly, I've killed her. Maybe she'll die in two days."
>
> She managed to walk home. But she was no longer really alive — she was empty: no blood, no life-spirit. She felt coldness coming all over her. Her head ached. She thought it was just ordinary sickness; but when she got back to her parents, she fell down, shivering and weak. Her husband came back with meat for them, but she couldn't eat any. They tried to give her food, but she wouldn't touch it. She lay there, shaking and moving restlessly in pain. They kept asking her what was wrong. Her mother held her, trying to stop her from shivering. Her heart was breaking to see her daughter like that. After two days, they felt the girl's pulse. It was almost gone. They sorrowed over her. With her last words, she told them she didn't want that man they had given her to. "But I can't talk, I'm leaving you now . . ." And when they pressed her to say who had done it, she told them, "He was the one." Her eyes opened, staring. They closed her eyes, straightened her body, put her legs together and her arms at her sides. Mourning and weeping, they covered her with a sheet of paperbark. Other men from that camp went to cut trees for a mortuary platform. They wrapped her body in paperbark. Her parents (and her closest relatives) were sobbing together a little way off, gashing themselves in grief.

The rest of the story is mainly a detailed account of the mortuary procedures and the people involved in them, with the girl's spirit answering her mother's soft calling; eventually, after the final ritual bone-collection, her bones were placed in a large basket for her mother to keep. But there is no further reference to the husband, nor any follow-up of the accusation against him.

In most such narratives, the storyline builds on three main features: cause, symptoms and outcome. Usually the outcome takes the form of identifying the "murderer", arranging for a running-the-gauntlet rite and/or killing the murderer or one of his close relatives in an open attack or through sorcery. In this case, Nganalgindja may have amplified the sections dealing with sorcery and mortuary arrangements, to make sure that they were understood — the approach often used traditionally in teaching children. As for the vengeance climax, she may have taken this for granted, implicit in the girl's accusation.

Margidjbu: "Powerful Men"

When we translate ***margidjbu*** as "native doctor", we use "native" as a neutral word meaning locally derived, of local origin. But because to many people it connotes "non-European", some other term is needed (see below).

Margidjbu appear in a number of myths, including children's versions. In a few they are central figures, but mostly they receive minor attention or none at all. One factor here is the way a storyline is shaped, and the aims and circumstances involved in telling it. In the three stories we have been looking at, no attempt is made to call in a *margidjbu* and no one raised the question of whether and how such a person could help. The last story was used conventionally as a warning to girls against upsetting the betrothal and marriage arrangements that had been made for them. For that purpose, the girl's death has a stronger dramatic impact than her recovery would have. The cave-painting story has obliquely the same implications, though the theme is complicated by the girl's readiness to accept other sweethearts — *but* those other sweethearts were young men, not old. This age discrepancy used to be a point of tension in western Arnhem Land, not only in stories (it is hinted at in the last one).

Margidjbu who appear in myth have "power" over and above that of most other mythical characters, even though all such characters often are assumed to have special qualities not available to ordinary people now. (The major mythical characters are in a special category in this respect, but are not usually called *margidjbu*.) In this region, women had a minor healing role, but the main *margidjbu* identified in myth and in everyday life were men. A *margidjbu's* feats vary according to the kind of story he is involved in. They included keeping the Rainbow Snake flood-waters at bay, at least temporarily; repairing and reviving a corpse torn to pieces by a crocodile (a meat ants' nest is the usual kind of life-stimulating agent); changing shape more rapidly than other characters can do; "feeling" what is happening at distant places; sending storms and floods to injure or destroy or punish people; or summoning his own personal magic-snake to protect him or harm someone else. A *margidjbu* can see ghosts and spirits, and other beings invisible to ordinary people, and travel in dreams more deliberately and more consciously than others can. Also, he is supposed to be more capable than other people, not only in coping with the risky sphere of the "supernatural" or extraordinary but also in knowing more about events and relationships in his own community. Ideally, he has both knowledge and "power".

One especially "power-full" character is Moon. The significance of his story is that it accounts, first, for the way the moon dies but returns to life after three days; and secondly, for the fact that all human beings must inevitably deteriorate and decay. (See, e.g., C. H. Berndt, 1964 : 272; 1979 : 15; Berndt and Berndt, 1964 : 397.) Even though Moon had "plenty of power", he could not help any other character in his story unless that character trusted him. There had to be a sharing, two-way relationship, not necessarily on an equal basis. This requirement was stressed in virtually all *margidjbu* transactions: nothing positive could be expected without mutual acceptance. That meant acceptance not only of the specific treatment but, as well, of the premises underlying it.

The same point was made obliquely in views about sorcery that were expressed in many myths and in discussions of them. People used to say that, even when there seemed to be an insoluble clash of interests, open conflict was not always feasible. But they used to say that secrecy and concealment in social relationships was bad in itself: it implied deceit and was potentially dangerous and destructive. Conversations in some myths, and in "real-life" cases, emphasized this: people were urged to bring whatever the trouble was, or their attitudes, or their secret actions, into the open. "Confess! Make it clear! Make it open, so we can all know!" The implication was that, ideally, mutual confidence is necessary for community well-being as well as for personal healing — for "good health" in public as well as in private relationships and activities.

In myth and outside it, *margidjbu* work within a predefined or pre-established framework. They are not all-powerful, especially when it comes to sorcery — which is another means of accounting for disaster, trouble and death. (See, e.g., C. H. Berndt, 1964 : 270–71; also in more general terms, Berndt and Berndt, 1964 : esp. 307–12.) A Maung statement summarizes the most usual fate of any person who becomes ill because someone has worked sorcery on him through his faeces or clothing or something connected with him (Lamilami, 1974 : 133): "He gets worse, and no one can do anything for him . . . The man gets sick, he gets weak, and then he dies. No one can do anything to help him."

More Specific "Do's and Don'ts"

Incidents and statements in some myths tell or remind the listeners about food. The ordinary course of events affords an opportunity for this, as the characters move about collecting food or hunting for meat, eating some things raw and processing others — or avoiding some things, either because of various taboos or because they "aren't good to eat".

In part of another story from Nganalgindja (early in 1950):

> Two Yiwadja brothers came south-east into Gunwinggu territory, making various creatures and natural features. At one Gunwinggu place, they met an old man coming from the south and the three camped together. He dug some bitter yams (*gubulurg*), a very "strong" variety, cooked them in hot coals and ate them. He

> didn't break them up first. [Nganalgindja added, "He should have pounded them up, crushed them, after he'd cooked them."] The two brothers noticed that he had tied some lengths of bush twine round and round his forehead, and asked, "What did you eat to make you sick?" he told them [i.e. he knew what he had done wrong.] After climbing up steep rocks with their arms about him, helping him, they camped, to allow him to rest. They left him in a cave while they climbed higher: he hadn't enough breath to go on. At the top of the escarpment, they practised throwing spears. One of the younger men's spears pierced the hard rock, and fresh water gushed out. The other praised him: "Is he a *margidjbu*, then, to do that?" When they climbed down again, to see how the old man was, they found him dying. They told him they had to move on — it was their destiny. "And perhaps you will die by yourself, because you found that sickness." [In effect, "You brought it on yourself!"] "But we have work to do . . ." He died later, in that cave, where his spirit remains today.

Some kinds of food should not be eaten, even after being processed. Lamilami (1974 : 32) mentions some jungle fruits that are "poisonous and would make you sick". For example, nuts or seeds in kurrajong fruit make a person's skin very itchy and lead to painfu sores. He tells a story of a disobedient young man who would no stop eating these seeds. When the itching became intolerable, he went into the sea to soothe his skin, and turned into a dugong. In much the same story, from the mainland near Croker Island at wha is now the Dreaming site of dugong (R. M. Berndt, 1970 : 18), the fruit affected the young man's eyes, "making them small and preventing him from seeing clearly. In pain, he ran down to the sea' and became a dugong.

Another example from Lamilami (1974 : 21) reminds listeners and readers that vomiting is not necessarily a sign of physical illness. Maiinaidj, fighting the giant Yumbarbar, struck the giant's testes, killing him. In an emotional reaction, Maiinaidj "started to vomit . . . shivering with fright".

Gunwinggu mythical characters — the First People, "they who were first" — did not like excess fat in their diet. In one story (Berndt and Berndt, 1970 : 45), "Two Yiwadja brothers who caught and cooked a large fish found it had 'too much fat, it made their hearts bad', and so threw most of the fat away uneaten." In another (C. H. Berndt, 1979 : 69), after a great wild dog had eaten a mythical woman, Aidjilad, "he began to feel sick". "His belly swelled up and up, from eating too much fat. He just crawled about in the sand, feeling very ill indeed . . . At last he died."

Several stories tell of "a great sickness" that spread over the land, mostly from the north coast, and how the inhabitants tried to cope with it. Before the final climax, when Moon's companion died (C. H.

Berndt, 1979 : 15), "They put sweet-smelling leaves on the fire, and tried to steam themelves better." Blanket (frilled) Lizard, in his story (C. H. Berndt, 1979 : 34), survived because he used red ochre: "whenever he felt weak he just painted himself all over", from his head to his feet, and "to stop his headache he tied round his head lots of soft, cold bush twine." This last is common outside myth, too: for example, cold inner bark from a banyan tree was a headache cure (Berndt and Berndt, 1970 : 38).

THE "REAL LIFE" CONTEXT OF MYTH

In the approximately three hundred western Arnhem Land myths and stories I heard, from the late 1940s on, many of the main themes and many of the details correspond quite closely to the case-history material and the conversations and discussions of actual events that I recorded during that time.

Conversely, not all of the local information about illnesses and their treatment is included in myth, even though it could be. Lists of "medicines" and other types of data help in building up a picture of the situation. Some songs are directly relevant too. Here is one example:

A Blister-pricking Song

This song is about prickly heat (*djaldjal* in Gunwinggu; *anaareen* in Maung), but the woman who sang it and the others present said it could refer to ringworm (*djilimin* in both languages), or to any outbreak of itchy blisters. The translation here is a general one, not itemized, given more or less as the singer explained it:

naréega wulga ya	She's sharpening a little stick, flattening it,
naréega mungiréebirée	Making it nice and smooth.
djeerin-djeerin gama	She's feeling itchy now.
budbud djeedawanei	She thinks, "How did I get this thing on me?"
buraa-buraa	It's getting bigger now, spreading;
marawein-marawein	Too many now, too much — those little prickly things.
nanáanganéela, nanáanganéela	(Noise of little blisters bursting, pricked with that stick.)

The song is not a mode of treatment. It is more like an irresistible response, an itch-relieving action taken almost regardless of whether it cures the complaint. No place-name was associated with it, and it has no specific "owner": "Anyone who has this prickly-heat thing can sing it!"

"First-aid" Materials

Some of the ordinary substances and techniques that people traditionally used on a do-it-yourself basis were noted in the myth-outlines: headbands of "cold" twine, liberal use of red ochre and steaming over a low fire of "sweet-smelling" leaves. ("Sweet" here is not the heavy sweetness, "like a corpse", which many Aborigines have said they do not appreciate, but a milder, more eucalyptus-like smell.) Hot ashes are a healing aid too. In the "sickness" stories, they are unwelcome, not in themselves, but because of the poison said to have been added to them. In the ordinary way, squatting over hot ashes or hot coals was recommended for relieving various aches and pains, and ritually mandatory in circumstances of childbirth and menstruation.

The range of materials available for treating minor illnesses and injuries was quite wide. Not all were mentioned in myths, although they could have been if a narrator chose to do so. Information about them was more likely to be passed on in the process of actually collecting and preparing and applying them, or in pointing out plants (for instance) growing at a particular place that people had gone to for other purposes.

In the late 1940s, people in the Goulburn Islands area were still using several products that were easily accessible and said to be effective. These are just a few. (It was not possible at the time to have them identified, botanically or otherwise.)

> For ordinary *sores* or small wounds, apart from red ochre, break some branches from a *yireelga* tree — a short shrubby tree with very small leaves. Scrape off the bark and boil it in water, making a reddish liquid, "like condy's crystals", and bathe the sores with this. Or, put thin pieces of heart-shaped *woràg-baràag* leaves on the sore, and keep them in place by tying with any of the creepers growing plentifully in the jungle. Or boil *baanggul*, a kind of mangrove bark (formerly used in trepang-curing), in water, then remove the bark, and when the liquid is just warm, apply it to sores.
>
> For *aching legs*, some people put their legs in water where they knew there were leeches, repeating the process as often as they thought necessary.
>
> For *coughs and colds*, one cure was a warm drink from green ants crushed in water. But there were others, based on a different kind of premise. One was a tiny shell, *yanili*, that women sometimes found while digging for yams. "Take it home. If you cough, put the spittle

into that shell, then put the shell on the fire, with paperbark in it to close it up. Keep on doing that, and your cough will dry up." Or do the same thing with a stone: "Put the stone on the fire; when it's warm, take it out, spit on it, and put it back again. Repeat until you are cured." A round greenish (unidentified) object found on the rocks serves the same purpose: *winyu-winyi*, the size of a football but quite flat, and soft and smooth with a hole in the middle. "If you have a very bad cold, coughing and coughing, spit into this; it will make a hissing noise. Then put it in the sun to dry up. You can use it several times; but when it starts to lose its colour, throw it away." (*Winyu-winyi* has another use: "If you have a sore on your foot, put this thing on it." But: "If you are walking on rocks, don't step on this — because, if you do, the tide will come up very fast!")

A full account of cures and treatments at this "first-aid" level would be very long indeed, and would show the same combination of straightforward empirically based procedures and others of a more obviously "magical" kind. The mixture of recognized physical treatment, *and* "belief in" whatever treatment has been recommended, is a small-scale example of a much more widespread state of affairs, and not only in Aboriginal Australia. It reflects the dual approach in the treatment methods of *margidjbu*, called in where more serious cases are acknowledged to be beyond the scope of "home remedies".

Sorcery Victims and "Abnormal" Behaviour

In the first two sorcery stories above, the cause-and-effect sequence is simply framed: the victims become ill and die, with no intervening event. In the third, the appeal to Nagidgid is believed to ensure that, for up to three days, the victim retains the appearance of being a living person. After that, he or she suffers the final and publicly visible misfortune. In this story, it was a sudden and fatal illness. Other accounts, mythical and "real-life", include a variety of ostensible "causes": snake-bite, a shark or buffalo attack, drowning from a capsized canoe, a fall from a tree, a spear wound, and so on. In local terms, they are not the real cause. They are only a screen, deflecting attention from what actually happened.

During these two or three days of living death, the victim behaves so oddly that discerning people begin to draw their own conclusions about what has happened, without as yet knowing who was responsible. The only person who knows is the sorcerer; but he continues to lie low about what he has done — "hiding his hand", in the Gunwinggu phrase. (A sorcerer always is assumed to be a man, though a woman might help by getting material from the victim.)

In the third story, the watching husband knows his operation has succeeded when he sees his wife eating a raw bird complete with feathers. This is the sort of thing living death victims do. They cannot discriminate between what is edible and what is not. Also, they are reckless to the point of irresponsibility. What they do depends on how the sorcerer has programmed them, what visible cause he has specified. For instance, they walk through thick, high grass where snakes are likely to be lurking, or throw away the paddles so that their canoe is helpless in rough seas (though only the stipulated victim drowns, while others survive), or go fishing in shark-infested waters, or make for mud-flats or swamps haunted by salt-water crocodiles, or deliberately provoke a spear fight.

Such breaches in the "normal" pattern supply circumstantial clues. Adults are expected to take reasonable precautions, to avoid dangerous places, to behave sensibly, and to follow the rules for living that they have been taught since early childhood. If they do not, the conclusion is that something is wrong — a something that is interpreted as "someone".

Abnormal behaviour along much the same lines is not defined in exactly the same way when it has been characteristic of a person almost since birth. A child who insists on eating dirt and pebbles and other inedible substances, and "won't learn", is distinguished from an adult who begins to do so suddenly for no apparent reason. The child's behaviour may be attributed to sorcery, but this is much less likely. More often, the reason is that either or both parents must have broken a taboo; or that a malignant spirit or ghost kidnapped the child temporarily, blocking his ears so he could not hear properly (therefore, could not "understand" and could not learn), and softening his tongue so he could not speak properly. Schoolteachers at Oenpelli a few years ago reported above-average incidence of physical deafness among school children; but physical deafness alone was not enough for people to identify a child as *bengwar* (Gunwinggu; female, *ngalbengwar*), "silly" or abnormal. (See Berndt & Berndt, 1970 : 156–57). There are only a few reported cases where a *margidjbu* was able to cure a *bengwar* child. In genealogical and other records, most seem not to have survived beyond puberty. Their affliction, however, was not referred to as sickness (Gunwinggu, *gundjag*) in the ordinary sense of the word, any more than the "living death" of a sorcery victim was.

From all accounts, in many cases *bengwar* children seem to have strained the resources and affection of their parents and others responsible for looking after them — so that the establishment of mission stations at Oenpelli and South Goulburn Island was seen as providing useful care and support centres for them, as well as for frail elderly and seriously ill or disabled people. There were enough of all these cases to suggest that local healing procedures either were not drawn upon, or did not succeed.[4]

The same conclusion seems to apply in regard to most sorcery cases, but from a different angle. The evidence appears to have been largely retrospective. "Why did so-and-so die? It must have been because . . ." And that concerns the identity of the sorcerer too.

The sifting of evidence, including interpretation of signs and accusations made by the dying or dead person (i.e. by the ghost), leads to certain conclusions. If someone is known or suspected to have had a grudge against the dead person, or a close relative of that person, the investigators have the beginnings of a case — perhaps the end of a case. A likely suspect might be a man whose betrothal came to a sudden end when the girl was married to someone else, or a man whose wife had rejected him in favour of a sweetheart, or one who had been rebuffed by a girl to whom he had made advances — provided enough people knew about the rebuff. Or the focus of attention might be a prior death. For example, "S.'s father was killed by a buffalo *because* he had killed L.'s father by sorcery." A number of cases were explained in such terms, in shorter or longer pay-back chains.

By the time a dying person was perceived as a *sorcery* victim, a *margidjbu* may well have been reluctant (in some instances, this was made quite clear) to take up a cause that was already lost. He might give reasons for being unable to take on a case: for instance, that it was "too late" for his healing powers to halt the process, or that revival of the "already-dead" victim was not feasible in that particular instance. In effect, a *margidjbu* could keep his credibility by not claiming to be able to handle everything, however difficult. In any case, it was up to the victim (before death) or the victim's relatives (afterwards) to approach a *margidjbu*, not vice versa. A *margidjbu* was not a trouble-shooter looking for people to help. They had to come to him, and usually recompense him with gifts for his services.

Traditional "Power" and a New Powerlessness

Western Arnhem Land was relatively rich in natural resources: in food, in water and in the materials people needed for the kind of life they had developed there — relatively, that is, in comparison with some other parts of the continent. Nevertheless, it is easy to underestimate the problems and troubles they had to contend with. Over and above ordinary environmental hazards, their expertise could go only so far in handling disease and serious injury or crisis. Their skills and interests and pursuit of technical enquiry were organized along different lines. In a difficult childbirth, for example, they did not have the empirical techniques to ensure a safe delivery. Major wounds and injuries and organically based illnesses were beyond the range of simple "first-aid" treatments.

Introduced diseases compounded their problems: smallpox (Foelsche, 1882 : 7–8, suggests it came with the "Malay" traders who used to visit this coast), leprosy, tuberculosis, venereal diseases, especially gonorrhoea, and in more recent times (for example) measles, influenza, the "common" cold and typhoid. They were even less well-equipped than Europeans to cope with such things, and far more vulnerable to some of them (measles and colds, for instance). Even a *margidjbu* "heavy with power" hardly could be expected to make much headway with these, in a setting that was increasingly dominated by foreigners with strange ways — almost as strange as *bengwar* behaviour, but with concealed power stronger than a sorcerer's. Traditionally, there were always limits to what a *margidjbu* could do — what he was believed to be able or prepared to do. In the changing circumstances, his abilities were inevitably affected. So was people's belief in them: strengthened in a few cases where they would turn to a *margidjbu* perhaps as a last resort, but weakened in others.

Opinions differ regarding the number of *margidjbu* in this region today, the power(s) they are believed to have or claim to have, and their current role. Collation and analysis of information regarding *margidjbu* and sorcerers in western Arnhem Land, such information as there is, has hardly begun. A lot more discussion is needed. However, several points can be noted in summary.

The "power" that *margidjbu* could use, power that came principally from spirits of the dead, was not equally distributed. Some men were believed to have only a little, some a great deal. Women could have "power", but not to the same extent: at least, no evidence to the contrary is available for the traditionally-oriented western Arnhem Land communities of a few years ago. Some women were adept at healing in the field of first-aid specifics: the whole range of getting and preparing and applying medicaments, and techniques such as massaging (as in childbirth). Also, women had the most consistent responsibility for preventing illness and injury among children: keeping them away from dangerous places and creatures, and dangerous foods such as bitter or strong roots that would make them sick; making sure their faeces were not left uncovered for sorcerers to find; attending on their behalf to food and other taboos — and teaching them to manage all these things for themselves as they grew older.

For illness and similar aspects, it seems that people did what they could within their own domestic sphere, where they had the resources and knowledge and precedents to handle an assortment of physical and emotional problems. If and when these failed, they might seek further help. Perhaps there is a near-parallel in the levels of advice and treatment provided either within a non-Aboriginal home or family setting, or by a chemist or pharmacist, or a general practitioner, or a specialist.

A "high-powered" *margidjbu* was more like a specialist. He could be expensive. Also, he was not to be approached lightly. Because he was believed to intervene between ordinary people and dangers of various kinds, especially supernaturally-based dangers, he himself was potentially dangerous. That alone was enough to set him slightly apart from others. But, although the most important religious rituals were concerned with promoting and sustaining *community* well-being, ideally it was the *margidjbu* who was believed to draw upon the religious dimension for the benefit of individual, here-and-now welfare issues. To do this, he had to be more than a physical healing technician. He had to be acquainted with the personal and interpersonal affairs and relations of the members of his community, and with its activities and ideas and ideals.

In a small-scale population with a more or less predictable range of expectations, this was a formidable task, though not an insuperable one. In the changing situation of the last few years, it has become almost impossible. For any *margidjbu* who are able to survive these changes, the definition of their nature and role must undergo (has already undergone) a fairly drastic reassessment.

This brings us back to the quotation at the beginning of the chapter — and the question of discrepancies in notions of health and illness, what these mean and why things go wrong.

In the Australian–European society that has been imposed on the western Arnhem Landers, as on other Aborigines, there has been and still is an emphasis on symptoms, on specific aspects (signs) of illness, disease, injury and the like — on specific physical manifestations, visible or inferred. In the field of mental illness, there has been the same individual-centred approach, although in the last few decades the concern with *social* psychiatry has been much more evident. The community health perspective has been slow to develop. Even now it is quite narrow in scope, although recognition of housing as well as hygiene issues has potentially socio-political as well as socio-economic implications.

This conventional pattern of illness and health also was imposed arbitrarily on Aborigines, as if it were traditionally their pattern too: as if their views of illness (and, conversely, health) were basically the same. But the views of western Arnhem Landers, for instance, were much more comprehensive. They certainly took into account, in their own way, the ideal of *mens sana in corpore sano* – but only as one small part of their orientation. Individual people were important but not as a narrow focus of health care agents. The western Arnhem Landers' concern was with individual persons in a much wider context. Their views about the transience of physical life as against the long-term continuity of spiritual life did not mean that they held physical life lightly – their own, or that of other people in their communities. (One matter in which their mythology does not "reflect" reality is that it is only in myth that people commit suicide.)

In looking over my information on this region collected since the late 1940s, I realized, much more clearly than before, that illness could not be seen in perspective without paying equal attention to the topic of health. "Health" is implied in the moral rules that are fundamental in sorcery cases, where answers are sought in social relations rather than in physical causes. It extends beyond that to the overall context, including the future-orientation, which for Aborigines (see Berndt and Berndt, 1978) was a guiding principle in dealing with the physical environment, with relations between people and with provision for oncoming generations.

Fears about the possibility of disaster following interference with the land, expressed in Rainbow Snake stories, have "come true" in the current scene, with the advent of large-scale uranium mining developments. Liquor has been another agent in this alteration of the Aboriginal lifestyle. The Aborigines' loss of independence has not been restored by the new nominal responsibility that has been permitted to them within a still-restrictive framework. Their understanding of questions of illness and health, and solutions to such questions, *must* be seen within the wider socio-political and environmental settings, and not merely at the level of individual or even intra-community symptoms and problems.

NOTES

1 Northern Territory Administration, Welfare Branch, *Annual Report, 1967–68*: 235.

2 See, for example, C. H. Berndt, 1964, 1979; R. M. Berndt, 1970; Berndt and Berndt, 1951, 1964, 1970, 1980; and Lamilami, 1974. My research in the region began in 1947, though I had worked with Maiali–Gunwinggu in army settlements at Adelaide River and Katherine in 1945. This contact has been maintained through subsequent visits and correspondence. All of my information came from women. (My husband's research was with men.) So much of the still-unpublished material of this research is relevant to the present chapter, that I have had to be drastically

selective: I have kept myth and case-material to a minimum. Apart from English, I used Gunwinggu as a *lingua franca*. Virtually all the myths, case-histories, etc. told to me are in that language, including such material in this chapter.

[3] In a different version, the island is called Gumur; see R. M. Berndt, 1970 : 35.

[4] The Methodist Mission staff at Goulburn Island kindly gave me access to the mission birth records (dating from 1918) and death records (dating from 1926). I went over these with local women, as a check on genealogical and census data, and also to discuss the recorded "cause of death", in the light of their views on each case. That led us into discussion of other cases and circumstances bearing on the subject of death, illness — and health.

REFERENCES

Berndt, C. H., 1964. "The Role of Native Doctors in Aboriginal Australia", in *Magic, Faith and Healing*, ed. A. Kiev (New York : Free Press of Glencoe), pp. 264–82.

—— (trans. and ed.), 1979. *Land of the Rainbow Snake: Children's Stories and Songs from Western Arnhem Land*, illust. Djoki Yunupingu (Sydney : Collins).

—— and Berndt, R. M., 1978. *Pioneers and Settlers: The Aboriginal Australians* (Melbourne : Pitman).

Berndt, R. M., 1970. *The Sacred Site: The Western Arnhem Land Example* (Canberra : Australian Institute of Aboriginal Studies).

—— and Berndt, C. H., 1951. "The Concept of Abnormality in an Australian Aboriginal Society", in *Psychoanalysis and Culture*, ed. G. B. Wilbur and W. Muensterberger (New York : International Universities Press), pp. 75–89.

—— and ——, 1964. *The World of the First Australians* (Sydney : Ure Smith; repr. 1977).

—— and ——, 1970. *Man, Land and Myth in North Australia: The Gunwinngu People* (Sydney : Ure Smith).

—— and ——, 1980. "Oenpelli, Then and Now: A Brief Overview", *A.I.A.S. Newsletter* (new series), no. 14 (September) : 38–49.

Foelsche, P., 1882. "Notes on the Aborigines of North Australia", *Transactions and Proceedings and Report of the Royal Society of South Australia* 5 : 1–18.

Lamilami, L., 1974. *Lamilami Speaks: The Cry Went Up. A Story of the Goulburn Islands, North Australia* (Sydney : Ure Smith).

Moodie, P. M., 1973. *Aboriginal Health*, Aborigines in Australian Society 9 (Canberra : Australian National University Press).

Northern Territory Administration. Welfare Branch. 1967–68. *Annual Report* (Darwin : Government Printer).

7

Psychiatric and Anthropological Interpretations of "Aberrant" Behaviour in an Aboriginal Community

David Biernoff

INTRODUCTION

Cross-cultural studies by anthropologists and others in health and health care have increased markedly in number in the last decade. Within this very broad area of concern, the uneasy marriage between anthropology, psychology and psychiatry continues, with cross-cultural psychiatry in particular being an active and growing field. As psychiatrists extend their interests further into non-Western countries and as indigenous psychiatrists are trained in the developing world, issues related to cultural relativity and ethnocentrism in the application of psychiatric diagnosis and treatment become critical. Can Western (or Western-trained and oriented) eyes appreciate the alternative subjective realities of those in other cultures? Is it necessary to appreciate their reality in order to care for the mentally ill? In this brief paper we look at these issues, with reference to a traditionally-oriented Aboriginal community in north-eastern Arnhem Land.

In the last ten years, a number of psychologists and psychiatrists have collected and published information from eastern and north-eastern Arnhem Land (see Cawte, 1976; Eastwell, 1973, 1974, 1976, 1977; Hippler, 1978; Kearney and McElwain, 1975). Relevant work from elsewhere in Aboriginal Australia also has become accessible (Cawte, 1972, 1974; Kearney *et al.*, 1973; Moodie, 1973).

Though some of these studies recognize the role of social control mechanisms in mobilizing negative sanctions against the "anti-social", none deals with the role of traditional structures and processes of social control that maintain and protect "land" and "law" in the subjective perception of physical and mental well-being. Thus although these studies provide useful data on personality and personality aberrations, they usually do not take into account the subjective reality of Aboriginal people. Nor do they explain individual situations and responses in ways that reflect Aboriginal understanding. The researchers' cultural and professional blinkers are understandable, but their reality does not coincide with the reality of many Aborigines in traditional settings. Aboriginal perceptions must be considered if valuable insights into the socio-cultural dynamics and health of traditionally-oriented communities are not to be missed. If cultural relativity is a valuable principle then the medical paternalism of many health professionals surely must be tempered with sensitivity and an awareness of cultural values and truths other than their own.

BACKGROUND

The field research for this paper was carried out over twelve months in 1971–72 at Numbulwar (mission) settlement, north of the mouth of the Rose River on the eastern coast of Arnhem Land in the Northern Territory. This settlement is geographically isolated and was, in 1971, little studied anthropologically. The only reasonable track led to the Roper River (Ngukurr) settlement, some 150 kilometres to the south-west. It was open seasonally for four-wheel-drive vehicles. Groote Eylandt lies just over 100 kilometres to the north-east across open sea. Yirrkala, about 250 kilometres to the north-north-east, is reached in two days by water along the coast. The only regularly used means of transport to other settlements and the outside world was by air, using scheduled or chartered air services. Bulk goods, including supplies for the store, arrived every six or eight weeks by barge. This geographical isolation provides insulation from the full impact of the European world outside. As a result, Numbulwar has retained a degree of cultural integration and continuity unusual in other Arnhem Land Aboriginal communities.

The central theme of this paper is the relationship between social control and "anti-social" or "aberrant" behaviour. There is strong evidence that hunting and gathering societies with low population densities and high mobility deal with aggressive behaviour by means of avoidance. When contact between people leads to aggressive reactions, one of the parties is expected to leave before a fight develops and someone is injured. Frustrations, anxieties or other sources of hostility thus result in a spatial redistribution of people, and residence groups are characterized by frequent changes in membership for the sake of peace. People who continue to behave anti-socially are ostracized. If they continue to be a serious threat to peace and safety, they are (or were traditionally) killed. This process effectively limits strife in daily life.

The Numbulwar settlement was established by the Anglican Church Missionary Society in 1952, to serve the needs of Aboriginal peoples along the eastern coast of Arnhem Land. Most adults had previous experience of mission life at other Arnhem Land missions, most often with Roper River (Ngukurr), established in 1908. Numbulwar was a traditional ritual centre, a focal-point at which many Aboriginal tribes periodically came together. Local Aboriginal peoples strongly encouraged the establishment of a distribution centre or settlement serving their needs close to their own "countries". By this time, after more than half a century of experience with Europeans on missions (and a lesser degree on cattle-stations to the south and on boats in the Gulf of Carpentaria and along the northern Australian coast), the members of the Numbulwar community had developed a considerable knowledge and awareness of the outside world, black and white. The isolation of Numbulwar allowed for the retention of aspects of traditional culture (for example, traditional religion continued to be practised, although in secrecy, since the missionaries disapproved, and the Aboriginal language was used as the vernacular for communication between Aborigines). Geographical isolation reinforced community pressure to keep alcohol out and minimized the impact of commercial interests and commercialism. Neither threatened the traditional orientation and integration of the community.

In 1971–72, the population of Numbulwar numbered between three hundred and fifty and four hundred persons, with two hundred and fifty Nunggubuyu speakers. Others spoke languages of adjacent regions of eastern Arnhem Land. As the dominant group at Numbulwar, the Nunggubuyu are the focus of study. They are divided between ten named clans, five in each of the two moieties. Strict moiety exogamy is the rule. At least twenty-seven distinct tracts of land are referred to by them as their "country". "Country" represents the main element in social, ceremonial and personal identity. Land rights and clan membership are inherited patrilineally through the male line. People belonging to the same "country" have common male ancestors and constitute a lineage. Lineages sharing common dreamtime or distant ancestors constitute a clan.

Prior to contact with Europeans, the Aboriginal inhabitants of eastern Arnhem Land subsisted as hunters and gatherers. The mixed environment in which they lived gave them access to a wide range of food resources, which were rich enough to allow considerable leisure. This permitted the development of an elaborate ceremonial and ritual life, occupying much of the time and effort of most adult males, and to a lesser extent, females. Studies have suggested that the dietary staples — mostly vegetable food collected by women — could be acquired in three or four hours daily. In the richer seasons, surpluses allowed more than two hundred people to camp at a favoured locality for up to three or four months. Major ceremonies took place at such times.

The Nunggubuyu mostly travelled within their own territory, between the Rose River in the south and the Walker River to the north, and inland to the foothills of the ranges. Occasionally they travelled considerable distances beyond this range, along the coast and along inland "roads", to attend major ceremonies throughout eastern Arnhem Land and as far south along the coast as the MacArthur River. Many adults came to be remarkably "cosmopolitan" after a lifetime of such travel and were able to communicate in three or more languages.

Normally groups were small. Large numbers of people only gathered together for ceremonies. Because people in residential groups were real or fictive relatives, social control mechanisms other than avoidance and rules that governed interaction between relatives were unnecessary, except in exceptional circumstances. Fighting and feuding between groups did occur, particularly over male–female relationships, but etiquette existed for dealing with these aggressive outbursts. Periodically, peace between individuals (and between groups) had to be re-established so that major ceremonies could proceed. Usually negotiations or peace-making ceremonies were conducted by the elders, who both organized the ceremonies and were responsible for directing the punishment of offenders.

Anti-social or abnormal behaviour that did not threaten the peace of the community usually was only the concern of the immediate family. For instance, persons incapable of caring for themselves usually were supported by their families, even though congenital deformities and mental retardation were sometimes said to have resulted from illegitimate sexual activity or breaking of food taboos by the mother.

THE PSYCHIATRIC INTERPRETATION

The psychiatric interpretation of aberrant behaviour in eastern Arnhem Land is succinctly put in the published works of Cawte (1978), Eastwell (1973, 1974, 1976, 1977) and Hippler (1978) and others (Bianchi *et al.*, 1973; Nurcombe *et al.*, 1973). More general statements and studies from outside Arnhem Land are presented by Cawte (1972, 1974, 1976). All of these are derived from studies of Aboriginal communities that utilize a research approach based on limited periods of contact with the community (e.g. Cawte's "short-stay psychiatric field unit survey"; 1972: ch. 1). Anthropologists generally have serious reservations about accepting results of research from periods of a few weeks or one or two months. They doubt that a depth of awareness, knowledge, insight and understanding of any human community would be gained in such a short period. Many of these studies thus are seen to be generally superficial, potentially projecting a view of Aboriginal communities that is distorted or unrepresentative. Certainly the statements and conclusions in these psychiatric studies do not seem to reflect the people (and their cultures) at Numbulwar, and elsewhere in eastern and north-eastern Arnhem Land.

Numbulwar has been chosen to illustrate some of the issues in the debate. The discussion below is derived from the author's own work (Biernoff, 1975a, 1975b, 1978, 1979) and that of Eastwell (1977). Although the material used in this paper is localized, the principles and issues revealed have a much wider application and significance within and beyond Aboriginal Australia.

The psychiatric epidemiology of the Numbulwar community is described in some detail by Eastwell. His study is based on twenty-eight days of work in Numbulwar, two days every six months over the seven years between mid-1969 and mid-1976. The author's own period of fieldwork at Numbulwar (1971–72) overlapped with two of Eastwell's visits, providing both with the opportunity to discuss impressions and conclusions at that time. Eastwell's epidemiological study is based on case-study work and a psychiatric and medical census of the community. Of twenty-five identified psychiatric cases, eleven were men and fourteen were women. The illnesses identified conformed to definitions used by the World Health Organization: "a case should be of sufficient severity to debar the patient from ordinary social life and work and . . . it should resemble some established psychiatric entity" (Eastwell, 1977 : 332).

Those of Eastwell's findings relevant to this paper can be summarized as follows: The psychiatric illnesses encountered at Numbulwar (with the exception of organic brain diseases) are reactive illnesses, resulting in a large part from the stress of living in the mission environment. Two psychiatric disorders predominated:

(a) *Projection:* "An ego defence mechanism whereby noxae such as sickness, injury, misfortune, or death [are] attributed to the malevolence of a rival clan." (Eastwell, 1977 : 338)
(b) *Identificatory or associative illness:* characterized by patients showing a similarity of symptoms, "often amounting to an identificatory imitation by the associate." (ibid. : 341)

Twelve of the twenty-five cases shared the excessive use of projection. There are three diagnostic categories of projection:
(i) Transient delusional state (fear of sorcery): The culture ac-

knowledges the existence of sorcery and, therefore, the community accepts that there is something real to be feared. If the putative sorcery is a delusion, it might be better to call it a collective, rather than an individual delusion. In the cases cited, the delusion and fear of sorcery always was projected outside the local group. Fear took no other form.

(ii) Dissociative reactions: The community believed that the patient's spirit had temporarily left the body, probably as a result of sorcery. This occurred at times of social stress.

(iii) Depression — and hypochondriacal complaints: These were seen more frequently after a death ascribed to sorcery and were thought likely to derive from a fear of sorcery.

Projection is an active part of the ideology of death, since adult deaths are believed to occur only as a result of sorcery. The clan leaders identify the clan responsible, which leads to increased solidarity within the affected clan, in the past leading to and requiring revenge. In terms of the psychological development of the individual, the child-rearing practices generate the acceptance of an external locus of control and reinforce the mechanism of projection.

Identificatory illness seems similar to epidemic hysteria. Most usually, siblings have similar and sometimes identical symptoms. The second sibling appears to develop the symptoms as the first improves. Culturally, the illness is related to very strong identity between siblings and by extension to other lineage, and even clan, members: they are the same entity. It is suggested that sorcery may be directed not to a single individual but rather to the (lineage) clan group as a whole. If one member becomes ill as a result of sorcery, the others also can expect to become ill. The ideology of identification also is seen in beliefs about shared dreams and telepathy, and is reinforced in beliefs about conception and practices of child-rearing, which result in the individual's identity being fused within a collective "clan ego". (Eastwell, 1977 : 342)

Eastwell (ibid : 343) concludes that the projective and identificatory illnesses encountered at Numbulwar "illustrate ego defences in the service of territoriality, reflecting spacing between family-sized bands and closeness within them. The net effect was to maximize the population that the band could support by hunting and gathering".

THE ANTHROPOLOGICAL INTERPRETATION

(a) General Considerations

We now will look at the cultural context of "aberrant" behaviour, using anthropological data: information that provides insights into the Aboriginal view of such behaviour. This data was obtained during a stay of twelve months and illustrates an orientation emphasizing the "cultural" rather than the "psychological". The information presented here was given by informants as part of the author's education into the culture of the community. In talking about illness, death and social processes, these Aboriginal teachers constantly emphasized the relationships between man, land and religion. Concepts such as social and personal identity, health, morbidity and mortality, anti-social (i.e. aberrant or abnormal) behaviour, law enforcement and social control, "spirit" power and sorcery, all were explained within a man–land–religion framework.

Ideologically, clan, lineage and personal identity derive from a real locality, an origin place that is the source of the "life spirit" and is shared by all members of an individual's lineage — past, present and future. Also associated with the origin place is an origin character — a dreamtime "hero" usually responsible for creating a number of related localities in various disparate countries. The deeds of these origin characters are related in origin legends. The legends provide explanations for the creation and distribution of plants, animals (and man), and many topographical features. They also give rules for conduct and provide basic models for social structure and organization. The origin ideology is expressed in ceremonial, political and social networks, and practices that tie the social and cultural systems together.

Individuals are obliged to protect their "country" and its sacred places (including the origin place). They must participate in relevant ceremonies, ensure that unauthorized people stay away from sacred sites, punish trespassers, instruct the young in ritual knowledge and practice, and maintain the secrecy of sacred places, knowledge and ceremonies. Those who are unable to meet these obligations and who otherwise break the "law" may be punished (as are trespassers) by their own or a family member's death or serious illness. Occasionally, fines may be paid instead. Punishment is expected even when an individual has no control over the situation, as when an unknown person (for example, a European) disturbs or destroys a sacred site. In such a case, those with obligations to protect the locality would expect to be punished eventually. The destruction of an origin place, since it destroys the life spirit of lineage members, is thought to lead to the extinction of the lineage. Legitimate punishment, that due to law-breakers and those who do not live up to obligations, is either directed by the elders of the community, or supernaturally, by spirit beings who reside at sacred sites.

The elders are the ceremonial and political leaders of each lineage. They direct the sacred life of the community. They are the repositories of sacred knowledge and traditions, including those for law enforcement. As judges, they are concerned with punishing law-breakers, those whose anti-social or aberrant behaviour threatens the peace and security of the community. The elders hold inquests, usually in secrecy, to try and determine circumstances and apportion blame and responsibility. Punishment, if required, also may be carried out secretly. The elders collectively hold the sanctions, the power and the authority to maintain control over all members of the community.

The above represents an idealized traditional system as portrayed by Aboriginal informants. It has been modified and driven underground, with an increase in secrecy, as a result of mission life and contact with Europeans and European culture. Informants claim that the system continues to function. However, alternative European ways and the settlement lifestyle have undermined the authority of the elders and increased resentment and ambivalence about their traditional powers and roles.

At Numbulwar, the establishment of the mission attracted people from different "countries" to come to reside together on a permanent basis. Where possible, they chose their camps or living-quarters so as to recreate the spatial relationships that had existed in traditional settlements (see Biernoff, 1979). In this way, people live in close proximity to close relatives and retain a social if not physical distance from more distant relatives and "strangers", who often are considered less trustworthy or more threatening. With permanent residence, avoidance or flight became difficult to use as mechanisms to minimize conflict. Other means therefore have come to be emphasized. In general:

1 There is continued belief in traditional social control mechanisms.

2 The peace-keeping role of missionaries, administrators and police is acknowledged.

3 A build-up of pressure (hostility and anger) is released periodically with public verbal abuse but little serious physical injury. (Combatants are restrained by concerned relatives and friends.)

4 Persistent trouble-makers are ostracized, with a threat of more serious punishment if trouble is repeated.

5 Close relatives feel that they are mutually responsible for each

other's good conduct and usually may be depended upon for moral, physical and economic support.

6 When the above mechanisms are insufficient to constrain conflict and the threat of serious violence between groups is real, the elders publicly harangue the community and insist on an end to the conflict. Usually this results in conciliatory discussions and the re-establishment of a state of peace (or contained conflict)

Contemporary Aboriginal communities exist in conditions of considerable stress, and this stress may affect the physical and mental well-being of individuals. But, importantly, the community itself is largely self-regulatory, taking advantage of existing mechanisms to retain its integration and minimize destructive conflicts. The Aboriginal community continues to provide a meaningful and fulfilling existence for most people. Most have a strongly developed and positive identity and self-image, and well-developed insights into the nature of human relationships, which make it possible for them to cope so well with the world in which they live. (These coping behaviours deserve to be studied in depth.)

(b) Murder, Sorcery and Social Control

The psychiatric orientation emphasizes the importance of the belief in sorcery. This belief often is said to create a very high level of anxiety in traditional Aboriginal communities. Such anxiety is apparent at Numbulwar, but it is rarely debilitating. Rather it is an awareness that (like cancer in our society) a potential threat exists. Sorcery is an intrinsic element in many Aboriginal cultural systems and as such is part of perceived reality. At Numbulwar, informants state that sorcery and murder take place both legitimately, as a means of retribution and social control (directed by "elders"), and, more commonly, as a means of vengeance by people living elsewhere, to pay back a grievance or to gain some advantage over the victim or his lineage.

The cultural system supports a number of beliefs relevant to this discussion:

1 The very young and very old die natural deaths. Other deaths are unnatural, the result of murder or sorcery.

2 Sorcery exists in many forms. Its effect is to manipulate and alter behaviour, and cause morbidity and mortality.

3 Sorcerers can be specialists or non-specialists. Both manipulate naturally occurring forces.

4 Distant groups have the most virulent sorcery and are most feared.

5 Many diseases come from dangerous, secret-sacred sites. They

are manifestations of the forces or power emanating from those sites. This power can be controlled and directed by some sorcerers.

6 Unskilled or uninitiated people also may release forces from a dangerous site, by disturbing the site.

7 (a) As sorcery is carried out in secrecy, no informed public knowledge of particular cases exists, except as gossip, hearsay and speculation. Public discussion is circumspect.

(b) Because of this secrecy, only an elder is likely to have access to information that might identify real and potential victims.

8 As retribution, sorcery is directed serially at members of a family or lineage. The serious illness or death of one member is followed by illness or death of others.

9 (a) Counter-measures may be applied, to identify the cause and source of illness and death. These are ritual procedures, referred to as an inquest, carried out in secrecy by a healer in the case of illness or collectively by the elders after a death. If the condition is a result of legitimate activity, nothing further should be done. Most often the condition is seen as the result of illegitimate acts by distant groups, in which case healing or sorcery may be used to counter the illness. If death has occurred, sorcery may be used to obtain vengeance on the responsible group.

(b) A healer should determine the cause of an illness, and should not interfere if it is a legitimate punishment. In such a situation, the victim should be left to die. A person attempting to alter the course of such just punishment likewise would become a lawbreaker.

Good health is associated with strict adherence to approved patterns of behaviour and avoidance of dangerous people, places and objects. A person's closest relatives, who protect and support him, secular and sacred objects to which he has rights of access and use, and localities known to be free from danger, by contrast, are safe.

As punishment may result from their actions, each person is concerned about the behaviour of close kin. One should try to direct and constrain them, to protect the family and lineage from risk. A healthy family has been successful in achieving these ends. It suffers no serious illness, and death only occurs in the very young and very old — except for those victims of illegitimate actions deserving retribution. The family suffering illness and death of previously healthy and strong members is seen as under attack, and at threat of further attack.

To the extent that anxiety and fear of sorcery can be separated from its more general awareness and acceptance, it functions positively to assure conformity to the approved behavioural norms. It also reinforces the interdependence and identity of family and lineage in the face of a potential threat of outside attack, and induces caution with unknown people, places and situations. Negatively, anxiety and fear can become debilitating in some individuals, who interpret illness and death as a sign of their own doom, despite support from friends and relatives. Traditional mechanisms may be brought to their aid. In the past, further attacks might be averted by:

(a) negotiations leading to conciliation and peace;
(b) amnesty, followed by holding a clan assembly or important ceremonies;
(c) exchange of kin, to create new kin ties between victim's and attacker's group (marriage and adoption);
(d) payment of substantial fines or compensation.

This then is the social and cultural context of "aberrant" behaviour. Many of the disturbances observed during 1971–72 could be understood both by Aborigines and by the ethnographer in the framework of social relations and social control outlined above.

DISCUSSION AND CONCLUSIONS

Psychiatrists and anthropologists appear to have rather different concepts of the nature of Aboriginal communities in eastern Arnhem Land. The differences have resulted both from different professional orientations and a markedly different approach to field research. Although there are areas of common ground, the emphases chosen reflect different philosophies and ways of thinking about human behaviour, the psychiatrist's concern being with the abnormal, the anthropologist's with the ideal and normal. Psychiatric research applies internationally recognized labels when trying to categorize observed behaviour. The underlying assumption is that those labels have universal application in human populations. It is asserted that each label is defined in terms of sets of observable symptoms. Individuals in any society observed to exhibit the symptoms, therefore, may be accurately identified as suffering from the condition referred to by the particular psychiatric label. While identifiable symptoms and aberrant behaviour do occur and are recognized as abnormal by both Aborigines and psychiatrists, it is not necessarily the case that labels can be applied automatically across cultures, particularly if they are assumed to reflect conditions that are both recognized and clearly identified in the culture. Thus the models for mental disturbance recognized in Aboriginal communities are almost never the same as those of the psychiatrist, especially if the Aborigines consider the behaviour as being an appropriate and reasonable response to a situation.

Eastwell's (1977) study attempts to take into account such cultural variables as sorcery and the close emotional links between members of the same family or clan, but it falls short of explicating the context and sophistication of these cultural variables, their logical place in the Aboriginal view of society, land and religion, and their positive role in maintaining (or restoring) group harmony and personal security. Does this matter? It is argued here that it matters for several reasons. First, societies are complex. Any scholarly attempt to identify and explain behavioural aberrations must be based on a sound ethnographic foundation, especially where the doctor-researcher and patient do not share the same cultural background. Whether or not culturally vague diagnoses are wrong, they are certainly shallow. Most importantly, they are a very tenuous guide to treatment.

Second, if Aborigines see some behavioural extremes as reasonable reactions to acute social stress (such as the imminent threat of sorcery) and others as real aberrations, it is useful to know for therapeutic purposes which category a disturbed person fits into. This will indicate when Aboriginal intervention may be appropriate, which conditions could be transient, which might benefit from medical treatment and which not.

Third, there are considerable physical and psychological risks in ordering psychotropic drugs for patients in remote communities, as is frequently done by visiting psychiatrists. Since specialists visit only once or twice a year and nursing staff or Aboriginal health-workers are left to administer the prescriptions, adverse and even irreversible reactions may not be noticed. (Eastwell (1978) notes such a case among his patients in another Arnhem Land community.) Treatment can exacerbate rather than alleviate the condition. These are reasons enough to encourage Aboriginal coping strategies and therapies wherever a "traditional" aetiology is suspected.

Finally, it is but a small step from explaining psychopathology in cultural terms, to describing culture in psychopathological terms. Eastwell has limited his study to the former, attempting to discern cultural realities underlying the disturbances of patients referred to him as a visiting psychiatrist and researcher. But it is deceptively and dangerously easy to assert that, if sorcery, shared identity and socializing processes are factors that emerge as central in discussions with Aboriginal patients and their families, these factors themselves *generate* mental illness. This is clearly illogical, if not absurd. One does not, after all, conclude in Western society that if one person in a family becomes emotionally disturbed, all families are a mental health menace. And yet, it is this very position — the assumption that Aboriginal society is sick and maladjusted by reason of its culture — that emerges in many other cross-cultural studies. This inference is not surprising in a profession whose concern is with psychopathology, but psychiatrists repeatedly paint a picture of Aboriginal communities as crumbling under the stress of the social environments in which they exist.

Perhaps the most consistently negative recent psychological description of an Aboriginal community is Hippler's (1978) description of the culture and personality of the Yolngu of north-eastern Arnhem Land.

Hippler's findings are at variance with the experience of all anthropologists who have worked with the Yolngu (including this writer). Those who have criticized the paper have noted that it is not only ethnographically and theoretically questionable, but is "negative and derogatory" in the choice of adjectives and phrases (Hamilton, 1979; Reser, 1981). For instance: "[By] comparison with western cultural norms, the Yolngu men are unrealistic and hyperbolic, the women concrete in their thinking and unimaginative ... emotionally impulsive and yet ... rigid in artistic expression ... These rigidities and lesser capacities are ... expressed ... in hysteric, phobic, counter-phobic and other defensive responses which are culturally institutionalized." Mothering patterns are "neglectful", "hostile, aggressive and careless" (see Hamilton's paper in this book for a very different perspective), and socialization is "impoverished". The results are "unconsolidated egos, splitting, unavailable adequate secondary narcissism [and] defensive grandiosity." The typical Yolngu adult is "an impulse-ridden, sexually anxious, jealous and fearful person". (Hippler, 1978 : 226, 237, 238)

Hippler represents a cross-cultural psychiatric tradition well established in Australia and captured by the title of *Cruel, Poor and Brutal Nations* (Cawte, 1972). As a reaction to this psychiatric tradition, many anthropologists discount much work in cross-cultural psychiatry. While not denying the stress and unfortunate conditions in which Aborigines live, they rather emphasize the stability and resilience of the majority of people, and their remarkable coping skills and adjustment to the world in which they live. Certainly in Arnhem Land, a high level of social and cultural integration, associated with strong positive social and personal identity, and considerable pride, is obvious.

Interaction within the local group is constant and intimate. It is characterized by a high level of support between friends and relatives, with personal interaction marked by affection, concern and consideration. Aboriginal people have considerable interpersonal skills, particularly in verbal and non-verbal communication. These skills are largely learned patterns of behaviour and formal rules of etiquette, based on a foundation of self-control and self-discipline, on the principle of reciprocal obligation, and on the ideology of sharing and mutual support.

The importance of the social network also can be seen in child-rearing. The Aboriginal child is born into a world of relatives in which the roles of mother, father, sister and brother, as well as other kin categories, are extended to a number of people outside the nuclear family. Thus the child commonly relates intimately with a large number of caring adults, who provide maximum support for the child. This reinforces the individual's identity and confidence within his local group. The varied adult models help the child to relate to and understand people as individuals, rather than measuring them against abstract ideals.

Given the many social pressures, the most remarkable aspect of Aboriginal communities in eastern Arnhem Land is that they produce so many well-integrated adult personalities, and that they provide people with a valuable and meaningful life. This is the result of features of traditional Aboriginal culture rather than a reflection of any new cultural behavioural patterns from Western societies.

It is against this background of social support and social control that the aberrant behaviour of a relatively few individuals can be understood, and in this context that their disturbances are most likely to be alleviated. Health personnel can thwart this process by practising medicine in a culturally chauvinistic way, or facilitate recovery by understanding and encouraging the traditional therapeutic social processes and coping mechanisms that exist in this, and other, Aboriginal communities.

REFERENCES

Bianchi G. N., McElwain, D. W., and Cawte, J. E., 1973. "The Dispensary Syndrome: Origins of Bodily Preoccupation and Sick Role Behaviour", in *Psychology of Aboriginal Australians*, ed. Kearney *et al.*, pp. 341–51.

Biernoff, D. C., 1975a. "The Dreamtime No More", *Current Affairs Bulletin* 51, no. 9 : 14–26.

——, 1975b. "Land and Law in Eastern Arnhem Land", *Occasional Papers in Anthropology, Anthropology Museum, University of Queensland*, no. 4 : 55–92.

——, 1978. "Safe and Dangerous Places", in *Australian Aboriginal Concepts*, ed. L. Hiatt (Canberra : Australian Institute of Aboriginal Studies), pp. 93–105.

——, 1979. "Traditional and Contemporary Structures and Settlement in Eastern Arnhem Land, with particular reference to the Nunggubuyu", in *A Black Reality*, ed. M. Heppell (Canberra : Australian Institute of Aboriginal Studies), pp. 153–79.

Cawte, J. E., 1972. *Cruel, Poor and Brutal Nations* (Honolulu : University Press of Hawaii).

——, 1974. *Medicine is the Law* (Honolulu : University Press of Hawaii).

——, 1976. "Social and Cultural Influences on Mental Health in Aboriginal Australia: A Summary of Ten Years Research", *Transcultural Psychiatric Research Review* 13 : 23–38.

——, 1978. "Mockery for the Ancestors: The Dynamics of Disrespect in Aboriginal Society", *Journal of Psychological Anthropology* 1, no. 2 : 211–20.

Eastwell, H. D., 1973. "The Traditional Healer in Modern Arnhem Land", *Medical Journal of Australia* 2 : 1011–17.

——, 1974. "Dilemmas of Aboriginal Marriage in East Arnhem Land, North Australia", *Australia New Zealand Journal of Psychiatry* 8, no. 1 : 49–53.

——, 1976. "Associative Illness Among Aboriginals", *Australia New Zealand Journal of Psychiatry* 10 : 89–94.

——, 1977. "Projective and Identificatory Illnesses among ex-Hunter-Gatherers", *Psychiatry* 40, no. 3 : 330–43.

——, 1978. "Supporting Aboriginal Ethnomedicine", written Submission to the House of Representatives Standing Committee on Aboriginal Affairs, *Hansard*, Friday, 7 July (Canberra : Australian Government Printer), pp. 2017–27.

Hamilton, A., 1979. "A Comment on Arthur Hippler's Paper, 'Culture and Personality Perspective of the Yolngu of North-eastern Arnhem Land: Part 1' . . .", *Mankind* 12, no. 2 : 164–69.

Hippler, A. E., 1978. "Culture and Personality Perspective of the Yolngu of North-eastern Arnhem Land: Part 1 – Early Socialization", *Journal of Psychological Anthropology* 1, no. 2 : 221–44.

Kearney, G. E., de Lacey, P. L., and Davidson, G. R. (eds), 1973. *The Psychology of Aboriginal Australians* (Sydney : Wiley).

Kearney, G. E., and McElwain, D. W., 1975. "Psychological Research in Aboriginal Australia", *Australian Institute of Aboriginal Studies*, newsletter (new series), no. 4 : 17–26.

Moodie, P. M., 1973. *Aboriginal Health*, Aborigines in Australian Society 9 (Canberra : Australian National University Press).

Nurcombe, B., Bianchi, G. N., Money, J., and Cawte, J. E., 1973. "A Hunger for Stimuli: Petrol Inhalation", in *Psychology of Aboriginal Australians*, ed. Kearney *et al.*, pp. 352–61.

Reser, J., 1981. "Australian Aboriginal Man's Inhumanity to Man: A Case of Cultural Distortion", *American Anthropologist* 83, no. 2 : 387–93.

8
"Bush Medicines": The Pharmacopoeia of the Yolngu of Arnhem Land

Neville Scarlett, Neville White and Janice Reid

> "We had our own medicine. We had doctors of our own — doctors who used to give a man life again. Now young people are giving that away. The old people have still got this medicine, but they're frightened to show white people. Why? Because of the mission. I'm asking the old people to show the young people how, a long time ago, when we were hurt, how to stop it — how to get up."
>
> Magarruminya, a Mardarrpa (Yolngu) man

THE PEOPLE

The Aboriginal population of north-eastern Arnhem Land has been referred to variously as Murngin (Warner, 1958), Wulamba and Malag (Berndt, 1955, 1965). While the north-eastern Arnhem Landers had no collective name for themselves, the word Yolngu (lit. "Aboriginal person"; cf. Balanda: "White person") has been chosen, after Chaseling (1957) and Schebeck (n.d.), since the earlier terms are confusing and the people now refer to themselves and other Aborigines as "Yolngu". The Yolngu, today numbering approximately 2600, occupy an area of about 26 000 square kilometres, bounded by coastline to the north and east, and river systems to the west and south. The climate is monsoonal and markedly seasonal. There is a wide range of vegetation types and ecozones, with the greatest variety on the coast. This diversity of habitats provides a broad and favourable subsistence base for the Aborigines, with population densities of up to one person per 2.5 square kilometres on the coast (N. White, 1979). The comparatively rich food economy and restricted movement in the wet season probably have been responsible, in part, for the considerable linguistic and genetic diversity of this region (N. White, 1978).

A substantial body of anthropological data exists on the Yolngu, beginning with Warner's *A Black Civilization* (1958). Much of this relates to their complex and controversial social organization (Morphy, 1978). The Yolngu language group, differentiated as it is into a number of dialects (Schebeck, 1970) — some so different as to be almost mutually unintelligible — differs in both structure and vocabulary from the languages surrounding it to the south and west. Within this broad cultural and linguistic complex there exists a network of genetically distinguishable units, which are closely related to drainage basins (N. White, 1976).

CONTACT WITH NON-ABORIGINALS

Indonesian (and especially Macassan) fishermen/traders came annually, and in considerable numbers, to the northern coasts of Australia, from at least as early as the eighteenth century (Berndt and Berndt, 1954; Mulvaney, 1969; MacKnight, 1972). Instances are known of Aboriginal men returning to live in Macassar (Tindale, 1925; Berndt and Berndt, 1954; MacKnight, 1972). Contact was most extensive in eastern Arnhem Land, where Macassan influence can be detected in the art, myth and ceremony, and in the technology and material culture of the region. Even though the Macassan trepangers last came to the area in 1907, Indonesian castaways, especially Tanimbar Islanders, continued to be blown to the Wessel Islands by the north-west monsoon winds (*Northern Territory News*, 20 February 1971). Canoes from New Guinea allegedly also have been washed on to the coast in the same vicinity (Mountford, 1956).

European contact in the north was spasmodic and temporary in the early nineteenth century and probably did not greatly disrupt the Aboriginal way of life, especially in the eastern Arnhem Land region (Berndt and Berndt, 1970). One of the main obstacles to permanent settlement, at least at Port Essington (1838–49), was malaria, said to have been introduced by the Macassans (Black, 1972). Palmerston, the present-day Darwin, was founded in 1869. During the 1870s, mining, timber and pastoral activities (with leases being taken up as far east as Melville Bay) led to increasing numbers of immigrants in the western Arnhem Land region (Berndt and Berndt, 1954). This led to a dramatic decline in the local Aboriginal population, due largely to the spread of introduced diseases, especially leprosy, which was brought into the area by Chinese labourers in 1874 (Cook, 1970). A number of mission stations were established along the Arnhem Land coast during the first half of this century, the first at Roper River in 1908. Like the mining camps and settlements in the west, the missions attracted Aborigines away from their own lands, into a new social and physical environment. Australian military bases were established near Oenpelli and Yirrkala during World War II. The 1960s saw the commencement of mining operations in the eastern Arnhem Land region: on the Gove Peninsula for bauxite and on Groote Eylandt for manganese ore. These centres have dramatically changed the lifestyles of the Aborigines living in the vicinity.

BACKGROUND TO THE PRESENT STUDY

The findings reported in this paper are based on field research carried out by the authors during the period 1973–80. Data on medicinal plants were gathered jointly by Scarlett, a botanist, and White, a biological anthropologist, as part of a wider ecological study of the Yolngu (see N. White, 1978). Information and plant specimens were obtained at Yirrkala (December–February 1973–74 and July 1974; the major source of information was an elderly woman of the Gaalpu dialect unit), Baniyala (Blue Mud Bay) in July 1974, and at Donydji, near the Mitchell Ranges, over a period of approximately eleven months between 1974 and 1980. Baniyala and Donydji are outstations established by members of the Mardarrpa and Ritharrngu dialect units respectively. These outstations receive a variety of introduced goods and services on a more or less regular basis from Yirrkala (Baniyala) and Galiwin'ku (Donydji). Reid, a medical anthropologist, spent twelve months at Yirrkala in 1974–75, with further visits in 1978, 1979 and 1981, in the course of a study of change in the indigenous medical system of the Yolngu. While her information on "bush medicines" was provided by several individuals, her primary informant was a woman of the Gumatj dialect unit.

THE YOLNGU TODAY

In most Arnhem Land Aboriginal communities today, introduced foods, together with changing settlement patterns and lifestyles, have led to discernible changes in health status. The extent of the cultural transition varies according to locality. For instance, Aborigines in the vicinity of Donydji outstation, while having a substantial and ever-increasing contact with Europeans, still base their economy on hunting, fishing and gathering.

From the Donydji study, and the research of others (e.g., McArthur, 1960; Meehan, 1977), it is reasonable to conclude that while there was seasonal variation in the quantity and quality of resources and times of undernourishment, Aborigines, like other hunter-gatherers (Neel, 1977; Truswell, 1977), procured a satisfac-

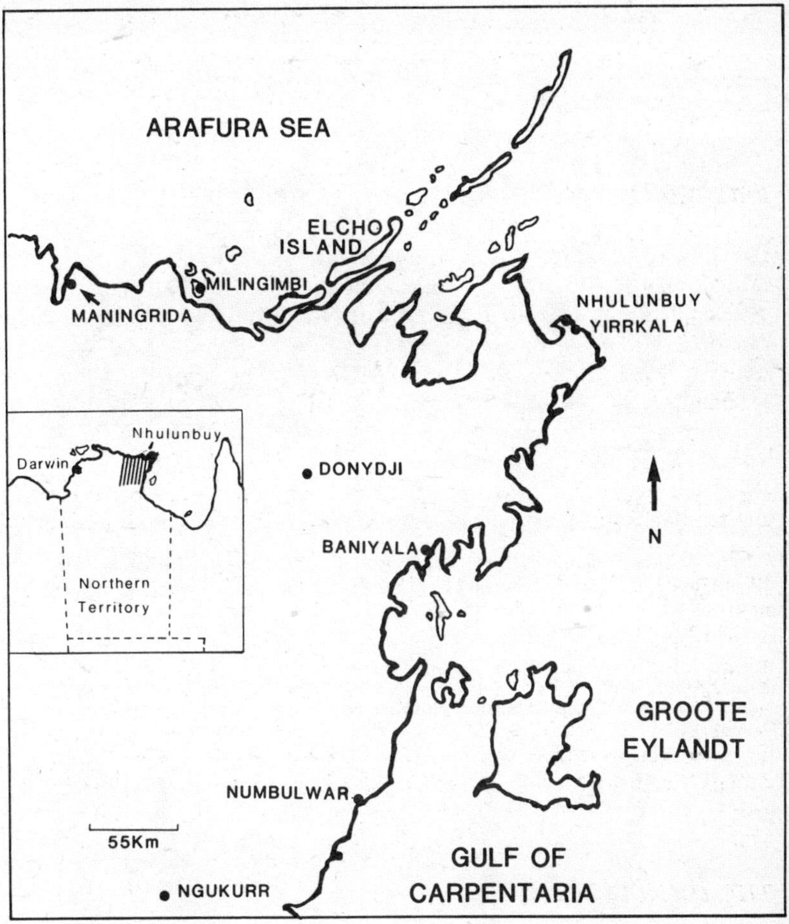

Map 4. Eastern Arnhem Land

tory diet without excessive work effort and with no evidence of nutritional deficiencies, even in the less favourable environments, such as the Western Desert (Elphinstone, 1971).

Aborigines living in the bush on outstations such as Donydji generally range over a smaller area of land than did their pre-contact counterparts and their diet is less varied. As the communities become increasingly sedentary, there is very often a deterioration in health, especially among the old and the very young. This can be attributed, at least in part, to their growing dependence on (and/

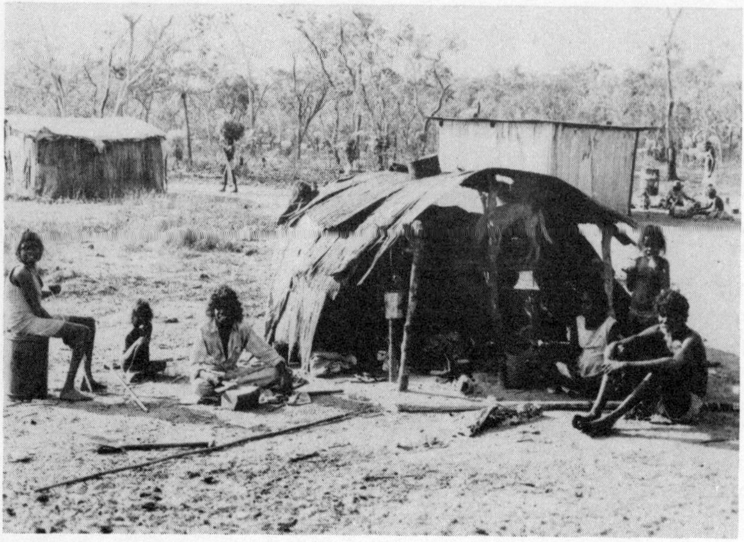

Household (Liadalingmirri Djambarrpuyngu ♂ x Gulungurr Ritharrngu ♀), Donydji, 1977; the corrugated-iron hut in the background (*right*) was occupied by single men.

Early morning camp in Birdingal Ritharrngu country, Donydji, 1977. The open woodland has been recently burned. Note the numerous cycad "palms" (*ngathu : Cycas media*).

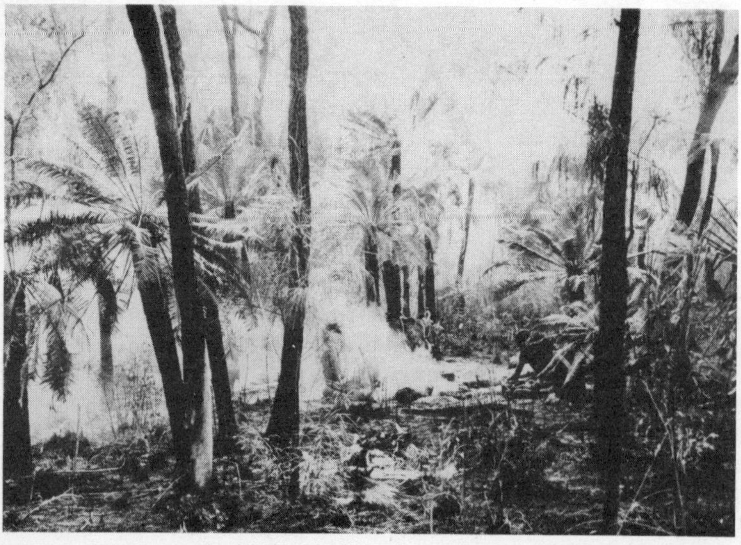

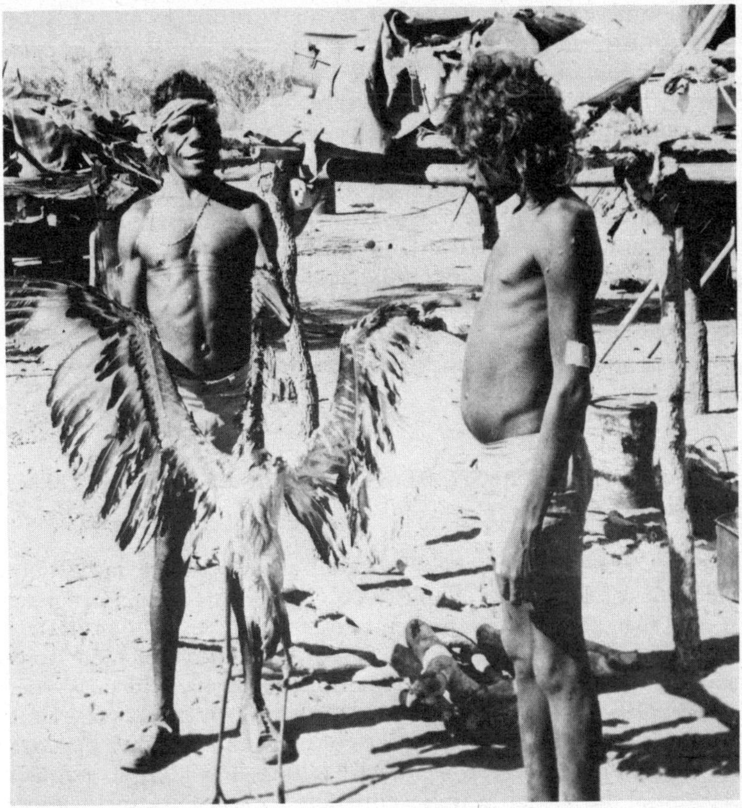

Birdingal and Gulungurr Ritharrngu young men with a jabiru (*gandji : Xenorhynchus asiaticus*), which had been shot for food; Donydji, 1976.

or preference for) introduced staple foods such as refined flour and sugar, as well as to the greater risk of infectious disease and parasite infestation. There is likely to be a substantial increase in nutrition-related diseases, as has been the case elsewhere in Australia (Wilson, 1953; Wise *et al.*, 1976). Here it is interesting to note that health data collected at Donydji and Yirrkala suggest that individuals living at outstations like Donydji have higher haemoglobin levels and lower blood pressure than their settlement counterparts (White, 1979). This is probably due to a healthier diet on outstations, based on bush foods. It also might be due to a reduction in lifestyle stresses away from the settlements, and in the case of the haemoglobin levels, less infestation with parasites, particularly hookworm.

There have been a number of accounts of the health of Aborigines today, and of the impact of introduced diseases on pre-contact populations (e.g. Cook, 1970; Moodie, 1973; Kirke, 1974; Taylor, 1977; I. White, 1977). It is agreed that in pre-contact times, the isolation, low population densities and nomadic lifestyle of Aborigines would have limited the establishment and spread of infectious disease. This situation changed following European settlement. Introduced diseases such as smallpox, leprosy, tuberculosis, syphilis, gonorrhoea, measles and influenza had a dramatic impact on the Aborigines. Doherty (1973) cautions, however, that some of these infectious diseases may have existed in northern Australia before white contact. Furthermore, there might well have been zoonotic infections, carried by native animals, that were important in the past.

THE STUDY OF "BUSH MEDICINES" IN NORTH-EASTERN ARNHEM LAND

The Reverend T. T. Webb pioneered studies of the indigenous medicines of the Yolngu people. Webb (1933) listed seventeen plant species that were used as medicines by the people living in or near Milingimbi Mission and gave detailed descriptions of their preparation and use in treating specific conditions. Lloyd Warner (1958 : 219–22) obtained related information from people of the same region (his "Murngin") in the course of broader anthropological studies. The Reverend Wilbur Chaseling (1957), in his popular account of the Yolngu people centred at Yirrkala Mission, included a brief but valuable reference to some common medicines that he observed in use. A botanist, R. L. Specht (1958), visited Yirrkala with the American–Australian Scientific Expedition to Arnhem Land in 1948. However, he collected little information on medicinal plants, his main emphasis being on species used for food and artifacts. Similarly, the ethnological list published by C. R. Dunlop *et al.* (1976) and based on their studies at Elcho Island (Galiwinku) contains only one plant of medicinal significance. Descriptions of some medicinal plants of Elcho Island, as related to a visitor by two women of the community, Djaypila and Yalwidika, are contained in the *Aboriginal Health Worker* (1979). Additional ethnobotanical data were collected from the Milingimbi area by H. Reeves, but this remains unpublished, although her typescript (undated) is filed with the Australian Institute of Aboriginal Studies.

Related work among neighbouring Aboriginal populations has been undertaken by D. Levitt and J. Waddy (see Levitt, 1979, 1981) for the Anindilyaugwa of Groote Eylandt, and by J. Heath for the Nunggubuyu, Ngandi and Ritharrngu, living at Numbulwar on the adjacent mainland. Heath's ethnobotanical data for the Ngandi and Ritharrngu groups have been included in his recent publications (Heath, 1978, 1980).

Results of the studies made by the authors are presented in detail in this paper's Appendix (pages 171–87), according to scientific name, Yolngu name and disease category. The proportion of herbal remedies employed in the various categories is further illustrated in Figure 3 below and compared with similar data from other studies in Australia and New Guinea. It can be seen that there is surprisingly good agreement among them. A further point in relation to Figure 3 is that Webb (1973) claims that a much higher percentage of species was used in Australia, in comparison with New Guinea, in the treatment of complaints such as coughs, colds, etc., and abdominal muscular body pains. He suggests that this pattern is related to the much greater abundance of aromatic sclerophyllous shrubs and trees in Australia. Recent data on New Guinea tabulated by Powell (1976) and summarized in Figure 3 do not support this regional distinction, however.

It is dangerous to extrapolate too far from the traditional pharmacopoeia in trying to reconstruct the causes and pattern of precontact morbidity, since there may well have been diseases for which it was believed no cure existed, and consequently no treatment given. This appears to be the case with corneal opacity and some snake bites, for instance. Given this qualification, the list of herbal remedies presented in the Appendix, and summarized in Figure 3, indicates that for the Yolngu, the common causes of illness were gastric complaints, coughs, colds, respiratory problems, wounds from accidents and fighting, eye, ear and tooth infections, headache, stings and bites.

While the bulk of the Yolngu pharmacopoeia is herbal, there are items of a non-botanical nature. For example, a white clay (Gumatj: *gapan*; Ritharrngu: *gurndirr*)[1] is ingested for the treatment of stomach upsets: a remedy reported for other parts of Australia, including Cape York (Taylor, 1977). *Dhalurunha* or red earth is applied to sores, wounds, chapped lips and sores in the mouth. Other exceptions include the bush cockroach (Ritharrngu and Gumatj: *buurduk*), the extract of which was used as an anaesthetic (see *burrpuy* in Appendix); a species of scorpion (Ritharrngu: *buthungu*), which was ground up and rubbed over the wound it made; a particular ant's nest (Ritharrngu: ?*garangaraykark/gangandark*) found in trees, which was burnt and the charcoal placed on "sore" eyes; crushed green ants (Gumatj: *galkal/ginilangu*;

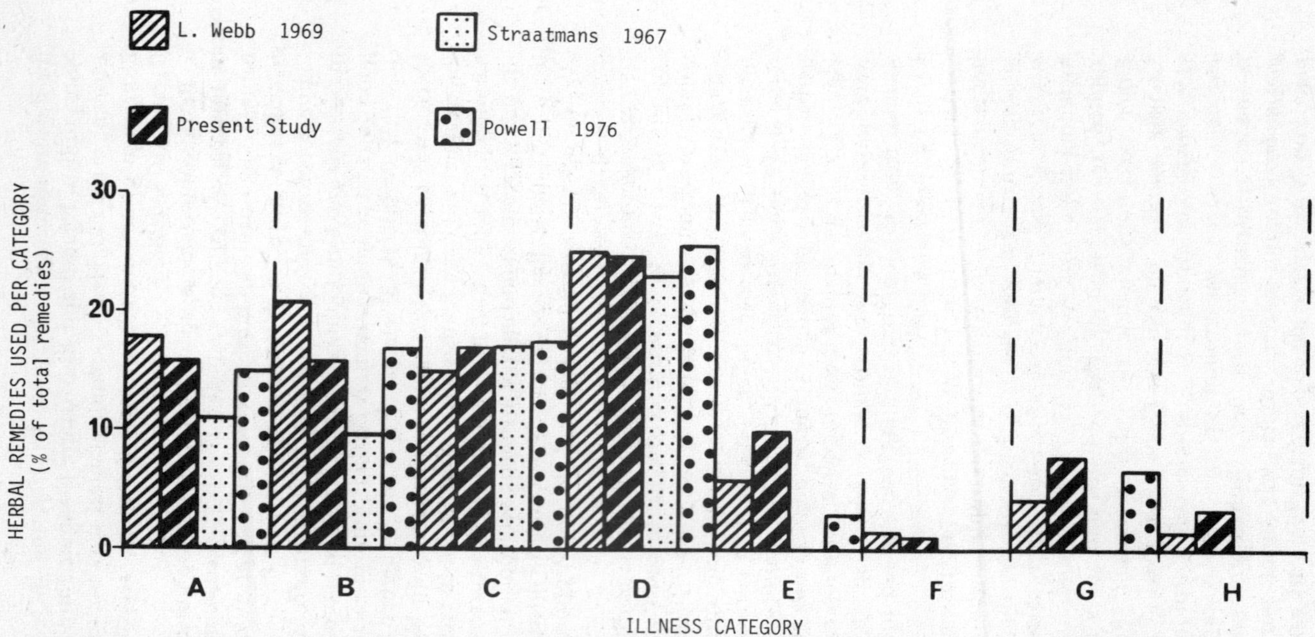

Fig. 3. Comparative Data on Use of Herbal Remedies by Indigenes of Australia and New Guinea, according to Illness Category
Note: The illness categories have been matched as closely as possible, but some minor overlap does occur. L. Webb (1969) used a questionnaire approach in an *Australia-wide* survey. The present study deals only with the Yolngu of north-eastern Arnhem Land. New Guinea data are derived from Straatmans (1967) and Powell (1976).

Code:

A Body pains and general malaise
B Cough, colds and lung complaints
C Gastro-intestinal complaints
D Skin lesions and wounds
E Eye complaints
F Ear infections
G Tooth infections
H Bites and stings

(adapted from N. White, 1979)

Ritharrngu: *malak*) used to prepare a lotion or an infusion taken for colds and chest complaints or as a component of other medications (e.g. *djiirri*); the brood-food (*dhurruguyag*) of a ground-living social bee, a medicine for lung complaints; laterite stone (Ritharrngu: *munmunda*), which was heated and placed on a sore and aching tooth; breast milk, which is used to wash the sore eyes and ears of children (see *barlkparlk* in Appendix); and *garrang*, a white "phlegm-like" substance obtained from coral, which usually is rubbed on the body for headaches, colds and influenza.

Taylor (1977 : 425), for the Thaayorre and Wik Ngantjera, noted that some bush medicines were "the exclusive property of men and their agnates". No evidence of this was found in north-eastern Arnhem Land, although certain plant preparations were said to be "women's business". These included plants believed to control fertility and lactation.

The scarcity of published data makes any detailed comparison of various "bush medicine" traditions difficult. Nevertheless, in an attempt to evaluate the efficacy or otherwise of plants used as medicines by the Yolngu, comparisons were made with information on herbal remedies recorded from neighbouring regions. The results are interesting. Of the genera represented in the Appendix, 5 are not found to the north of Australia, with only 2 genera truly endemic: 36 closely related or identical species to those listed are found in the Indo-Malaysian region. Of these, 32 (89 per cent) are put to similar medicinal use (based on Burkill, 1966). This correspondence can be interpreted in a number of ways: (a) the store of knowledge came with the early immigrants from the Indo-Malaysian region, ancestors of present-day Yolngu; (b) the herbal remedies were discovered in the two regions independently (providing support for their medicinal efficacy); (c) the Yolngu acquired knowledge of the use of these plants from historically recent voyagers to northern Australia, especially from the Macassans. The first hypothesis receives support from Golson (1971 : 199), who demonstrated a similarly high correspondence for food plants in the Arnhem Land and Malaysian regions. He concluded that at the "generic or specific level . . . the vast majority of the plants used for food in Arnhem Land would have been familiar to immigrants from the Malaysian region."

There is no doubt, however, that medicinal plants were of common interest to both the Macassans and the Yolngu. Lloyd Warner's main informant, Mahkarolla, in describing his childhood, talks of Yolngu (specifically Wangurri) giving Macassans "pearl shell, pearls, tortoise shell, sandalwood, and other woods they use[d] for medicine" (Warner, 1958 : 568). Such medicines probably were of interest not only to the Macassans but also the Chinese, with whom they traded. Furthermore, Burkill (1966) refers to sailors of Macassar taking fruits and roots of at least one medicinal species (*Clerodendron* sp.) to sea with them. In this case, one of a number, the medicinal use to which the plant was put was identical in Indonesia and north-eastern Arnhem Land, namely as a tonic for the treatment of "stomach upsets" (see Appendix).

Additional support for the contention that knowledge of medicinal plants was exchanged between the Yolngu and Macassans is provided by the following comparative data, based on published accounts of plant medicines used by the indigenes of Queensland (L. Webb, 1969) and New Guinea (Straatmans, n.d., and 1967; Powell, 1976). The data can be summarized as follows: In northern Queensland can be found 44 of the same, or closely related, species documented by Scarlett *et al.* (this paper) for the Yolngu. However, in this region of Aboriginal Australia, only 8 species (18 per cent) are recorded by Webb (1969) as having been used for the same purpose. In fact, based on Webb, 27 (61 per cent) common or related species were not listed as Aboriginal plant medicines. There was a slightly greater correspondence between the north-eastern Arnhem Land use of plant medicines and the New Guinea material. Here 23 species are found in common with north-eastern Arnhem Land. Of these, 9 (39 per cent) are reported by Straatmans and/or Powell as having a similar use, while 8 (35 per cent) are not listed as having been used. The published data of Webb are certain to be incomplete, derived as they are from questionnaire material, and more extensive surveys in the Cape York region may modify the picture significantly. Here it is interesting to note that the 8 north-eastern Arnhem Land "medicinal" species/genera found in central Australia are all employed medicinally in that region (P. Latz, pers. comm.)

The findings for the Yolngu are in agreement with Taylor (1977 : 425) who in his study of a "pre-contact Aboriginal medical system" on Cape York Peninsula, noted that "some of the bush medicines were symptom specific and were widely known", such as the treatments for sore eyes, colds and diarrhoea. "Other treatments were more general in their application and could be described as all-purpose remedies." The Ritharrngu, for example, use *Clerodendron floribundum* (*walpurrunggu'-ngining*) externally in the treatment of sores, cuts, body pains and general malaise, and internally for coughs, colds, chest complaints, gastro-intestinal problems and general aches and pains. Conversely, in the treatment of specific illnesses or injuries, medical agents were sometimes non-specific. For instance, when a person was "stung" by a particular caterpillar (*dhapalany*), he took any leaf, heated it and rubbed it on the "sting".

The problem that arises with any evaluation of the efficacy of a traditional medical system is the level of causation posited by the people, and whether the treatment is "natural" or "supernatural" (in Western terms). For instance, at Donydji in 1976, during a time of considerable social tension following a clan dispute, a message came to the camp that a young Ritharrngu man had "cut his foot off". With a great deal of apprehension, and armed with a small and very inadequate medical kit, we set off to provide first-aid. On reaching the injured person, who appeared to be greatly distressed, it was found he had suffered only a minor foot wound caused by a splinter of wood. Upon removal of the splinter and treatment with antiseptic cream and a band-aid, the "patient" was ceremoniously carried the three kilometres back to camp in a wheelbarrow. The next evening he participated in a *buku'lup*, or ritual purification ceremony.

In this case people's interest was centred on the "ultimate" cause of the injury — believed to be sorcery — though there was no denying that the approximate cause was the splinter. An indication of the level of anxiety in the community was evident from the extent of exaggeration of the wound: the worst was expected. Examples such as this confirm the view that in Aboriginal society "good health has ultimately to do with good social relationships" (Bell, 1978 : 4).

Nevertheless, more extensive research, including chemical analyses, is needed on Aboriginal herbal medicines to evaluate their therapeutic properties. Some of the more specific remedies especially are likely to be of medicinal value, for as Webb (1969 : 139) concludes from his continent-wide survey, "The convergence of use of the same species in different localities, and the survival of the reputation of alleged remedies, provide some circumstantial evidence in favour of the efficacy of such species." Other remedies of a less-specific nature and those obviously magical were probably ineffective at the biological level. However, these, like the Aboriginal healer, may have exerted a positive effect of a psychological or social nature.

THE TRADITIONAL MEDICAL SYSTEM

The Yolngu see a harmony between man and the endless cycle of nature, within which there is no clear distinction between the natural and the supernatural. This notwithstanding, ethnographers and anthropologists appear to have overemphasized the supernatural aspect in the Aboriginal understanding and explanation of well-being, illness and death. Conversely, the recognition of natural causes for illness and injury probably has been understated. Certainly recent investigations (by N. W.) at Donydji show that there is an acknowledgement of the relationship between physical cause and biological consequence in the area of health and well-being. For instance, diet and weather are both seen to be ultimately related to health. Examples of this naturalistic view of illness include: "wet" sores (*djeli'*), said to be caused by excessive sweating (*wulburr*), especially when sleeping in a hot place without a breeze; sores (*djidji*, *mapay*), caused by wounds from grass etc. or burns; coughs and lung complaints, attributed to being "slack inside" as a consequence of a diet deficient in meat; diarrhoea (*birlbirlgu*), which, it is said, can be caused by dietary factors such as vegetable food that is "too dry" (*barndany*), cycad bread (*munbuwa*) made from old nuts, and *Dioscorea transversa* (*ganguri*) eaten at the wrong time of the year; and headaches (*rathala*) resulting from "dry" food or excessive exposure to the sun. Ritharrngu say that if you "want to feel good" (*djaalngamadhirri*), you should eat a mixed diet (*miilmarnabarn*), a diet of meat and vegetable food. In fact, these two words often are used interchangeably.

Such observations, together with a quite detailed lexicon of anatomical terms, are inconsistent with the view that Aboriginal medicine focused only on the supernatural, denying the purely natural origins of disease. It cannot be denied, however, that sorcery and supernatural agents form an important, possibly *the* most important, component of the Yolngu view of illness and death. For example, Ritharrngu male informants have attributed the symptoms of yaws and leprosy to sorcery, and corneal opacity (*miilbaruna*) to the breaking of food taboos. Diarrhoea in some cases was treated magically: by prodding the excrement with bark or sharp sticks. Similarly, string made from *Brachychiton paradoxum* (Ritharrngu: *barlgurr*), when placed on a spear wound for instance, makes a man "wake up and walk". (A detailed description of Yolngu beliefs about the non-natural causes of illness, particularly sorcery and spirits, is contained in Reid, 1978b.)

THE USE OF "BUSH MEDICINES" IN THE SOCIAL CONTEXT

The healing role in Yolngu society, and indeed in Aboriginal society as a whole, has been discussed in greatest detail by anthropologists in reference to the "medicine men" or Aboriginal doctors (Gumatj: *marrnggitj*; Ritharrngu: *girlipa*; *garlang*). The powers and abilities of Yolngu doctors have been amply documented (Eastwell, 1973; Reid, 1978a; Thomson, 1961; Warner, 1958; T. Webb, 1936). Research in north-eastern Arnhem Land suggests, however, that the emphasis placed on the healing powers of Aboriginal doctors in the literature may belie the frequency with which they were and are actually consulted.

The spiritual healer does not use herbal treatments in his practice; he is a specialist who operates primarily at the spiritual and social levels. As in other areas of Australia (Cawte, 1974; Elkin, 1977), his ability to cure comes from the possession of spiritual powers or of powerful objects given to him by spirit-beings. Whereas any person may learn to identify, prepare and use "bush medicines", the Aboriginal doctor is a specialist who has exceptional knowledge and powers. As such, he is only called upon to treat serious or chronic illness that does not respond to the usual medications, which any person can administer. No more than one or two people in a community would be recognized as *marrnggitj*. By contrast, every adult and many older children would know of at least a few "bush medicines". The older women especially collected and prepared herbal remedies. This is not to deny that men have, or use, this knowledge. It suggests that the women are as important, if not more so, in providing the link between the Western medical system and the traditional system — at least on the practical side in the distribution and application of medicines.

The significance of "bush medicines" in the treatment of illness in the period before European contact can be appreciated by studying present-day choices for treatment offered to sick people and their families. In contemporary Yirrkala, people have several choices when they fall ill. They may, as often happens, simply bear the pain and discomfort, in the hope that the condition will be self-terminating. However, when it becomes clear that an illness is lingering or is causing sufficient discomfort to warrant treatment, action is taken.

First, the sick person may self-medicate or may be give medicine by a family member, usually a mother or wife. These days "cough medicines", "aspro" and "rubbing medicine" are popular and are available from the community store at Yirrkala or from the pharmacy in the nearby mining-town of Nhulunbuy. Occasionally women will produce from storage old bottles of pills or eye and ear drops and administer these.

If home treatment, or simply waiting for an illness to pass, does not seem to be working, the sick person usually will seek treatment from the staff of the community health centre. At Yirrkala, the centre is staffed by Aboriginal health workers. Each week-day morning, adults and children attend the clinic, seeking treatment for injuries, upper respiratory tract infections, gastro-enteritis, eye and ear infections, skin conditions, headaches, urogenital infections and other common illnesses. If the staff, patient or family consider that the illness is sufficiently serious to warrant further medical examination and treatment, the patient will be taken to Nhulunbuy Hospital or visited by the doctor on his weekly rounds. In rare cases, patients are flown to Darwin or to southern hospitals for treatment not available in the region (such as certain surgical procedures or radiotherapy). If family members consider that the illness is intractable, serious or life-threatening, they may also request the services of the *marrnggitj*. He (or she) is normally consulted during the latter stages of an illness, when it has become clear to the patient and his family that other options have failed and when they begin to suspect an underlying cause, such as sorcery or the actions of spirits.

On outstations, the sequence of events is similar, but the final recourse to the nearest health centre or hospital is taken with greater reluctance, since it involves evacuation by road or air, separation from one's family and the possibility of dying away from one's country (see N. White, 1978).

It is reasonable to assume that, prior to the coming of Europeans, herbal medicines would have been used, as Western medicines are today, in the early stages of the search for a cure for an illness. Wives, mothers or sisters would have collected, prepared and administered herbal remedies to sick members of their families. Their role in medical treatment today has substantially been assumed by the health personnel who have the major responsibility for attending to illnesses and injuries that are not critical. On large settlements such as Yirrkala, the health centre staff are in many ways the latter-day equivalent of the traditional female herbalists of each family. Similarly, the common Western pharmaceutical preparations that health centre staff have at their disposal are the functional equivalents of Yolngu "bush medicines". At Yirrkala, critical illnesses are referred to the doctor at Nhulunbuy Hospital, much as serious conditions were (and in some cases still are) referred to *marrnggitj* under the Yolngu system of medical care.

With access to a wide range of Western medicines and treatments, the use of "bush medicines" today is decreasing. Normally they are used now as an occasional adjunct to Western medicine, not as an alternative. Of 43 people at Yirrkala from whom personal medical histories were elicited, only half (22) had used bush medicines at some time (or been treated with them by a female relative, usually a mother). There was no significant difference between the younger (under thirty years of age) and older (over thirty years) age groups in this respect. At Donydji, however, most people had used, and many were using, traditional medicines. Again, there appeared to be no age effect in this respect, although apparent differences in attitude between the younger and older groups were noted in the use of the "cleansing" or "purification" ceremony, known as the *buku'lup* (lit. "forehead washing"). Unlike the older informants spoken to in this context, some younger males claimed the *buku'lup* could be used in the treatment of illness.

Although "bush medicines" are used infrequently, no one consulted expressed doubts about their effectiveness. They are still well known and enthusiastically listed by many adults as a unique asset of their own society. A conversation that took place at Donydji in April 1980 illustrates this. "Our medicine is better for this sickness than yours", said Dhulutarama, an elderly Birdingal Ritharrngu man, who was complaining of a chest infection and associated fever. To the question: "Then why not use it now, instead of asking me for aspirin and cough mixture?", he immediately answered: "Because you're here!" Is it true that the traditional remedies known to Dhulutarama are more effective in the treatment of his medical condition — or was it a matter of pride; a need to reassert his own beliefs and cultural values in the face of ever-increasing Western influence, while recognizing that Western medicines were preferable to his own? Perhaps, as he implied, it *was* simply a matter of convenience, in that here were medicines he was familiar with, while traditional treatment required the collection of plants that were not readily available and that required considerable time and effort to prepare.

None the less, there has been a dramatic loss of traditional knowledge of bush medicines among the young in large communities such as Yirrkala. In fact, this is true of ethnobotany in general. Just as in the case of Dhulutarama, the dwindling use of "bush medicines" appears to lie, not in a lack of faith among community members in their efficacy, but in the difficulties and costs of obtaining them. The health centre at Yirrkala is a comparatively short walk away, and it is easier to go there first seeking care when the medicines it provides are generally acknowledged to be effective for most conditions.

Those who would like to use "bush medicines" are, perhaps, more discouraged by the realization that the overwhelming majority of illnesses that they now experience are not indigenous (or that their high prevalence defies home treatment) and therefore must be combated with non-indigenous medicines. For instance, since the early 1970s, many cases of acute fish poisoning have occurred among European and Aboriginal residents at Nhulunbuy and Yirrkala. The Aboriginal sufferers and their families declare that fish poisoning (identified by medical authorities as ?*Cigatuera* sp. poisoning) was unknown in these waters until the bauxite mine and processing plant was established in the late 1960s. Many attribute the condition to toxic wastes flowing into the sea from the plant. Others, including local Whites, blame changes to the seafloor ecosystem caused by bauxite dust. One woman who was concerned that she or her family might eat poison fish while living at an off-shore island outstation, was asked whether she could not use the local "bush medicines". She gave a withering look and said that fish poisoning was a sickness caused by Europeans and therefore needed European medicine. Her opinion was not shared, however, by everyone. Another woman attempted to treat herself with *gawurlurr-nganing* after she had eaten poison fish, but also went to the health centre, in the hope that at least one of the medications would work. Similarly, although measles is an introduced disease, one mother said she treated her child with *muthi* when he contracted the disease.

Although "bush medicines" are not used often at Yirrkala, middle-aged and older women can not only name but locate, describe and prepare these medicines. The health workers themselves are conversant with "bush medicines", and on at least three occasions known used certain plants (*nhaambarra*, *maanyarr* and *girrigirri*) in conjunction with Western preparations. Older men also are familiar with most "bush medicines", though they are less inclined to spend time detailing their names and uses or gathering and administering them.

"Bush medicines" can be seen, then, as constituting a relatively dormant segment of an extended pharmacopoeia that includes Western and Aboriginal preparations. Generally they are used today only when they are handy and when Western medicines are not, or when Western medicines have proved to be ineffective. This is particularly the case for people living at remote outstations. Two clan and outstation leaders stated independently that "bush medicines" are used more often when people are away from Yirrkala, especially when the supply of medicines left by Department of Health staff runs out. This was confirmed by observations at Donydji and Baniyala.

It seems reasonable to assume that, as with other cultural practices that have been revived when people have "gone home" (as some describe the return to traditional territories), "bush medicines" will increase in favour and use. It also seems likely that the knowledge possessed by the older women and men about their properties and preparation will be passed on to the young as they watch them being collected and used. This trend is likely not only because people are farther away from Western medical services, but because, in reasserting their independence from European service structures, outstation dwellers are regaining a sense of control of their own lives, which predisposes toward Aboriginal ways of handling crises, be they social or medical.

ACKNOWLEDGEMENTS

The studies reported above could only have taken place with the co-operation of the various Aboriginal communities. In particular, we wish to thank those people who gave their support and friendship. They include Banguyarri, Milminyina, Laklak, Bakamana, Djuwandayngu and Bakali at Yirrkala; Gurruwul, Milwathayn and Djaapari at Baniyala; and the entire Donydji community, especially Dhulutarama, Dhanggarlgarl and Yilarama.

Many of the observations reported in this paper were recorded during fieldwork studies supported by the Australian Institute of Aboriginal Studies, for which we are grateful.

We also gratefully acknowledge the work of M. Forrester in co-ordinating and typing a difficult manuscript and M. McDowall for preparing the artwork.

Dr K. Semmens provided valuable comments on the manuscript. N. W. wishes to thank Peter Latz, and also Professor J. Golson for helpful discussion and the opportunity to research and prepare aspects of this paper while a Visiting Fellow in the Department of Prehistory, Research School of Pacific Studies, Australian National University. J. R. is grateful to Ms Alison Stefanska of the Northern Territory Department of Health, for arranging the identification of her collection of Yolngu "bush medicines".

Appendix[2]

MEDICINAL PLANT SPECIES OF NORTH-EASTERN ARNHEM LAND

Notes:

a Nomenclature mainly follows Chippendale, 1971. In cases where nomenclature differs, the appropriate authorities are cited.

b Records from Yirrkala, Baniyala and Donydji are denoted by Y, B and D, respectively.

c Numerals shown in parentheses indicate the reporting authority, namely: (1) W. Chaseling, (2) J. Reid, (3) N. Scarlett, (4) R. Specht (1958), (5) L. Webb (1969), (6) T. Webb (1933), (7) N. White.

d The Yolngu name of the plant is given following the Western scientific name.

Alphitonia petrei (Rhamnaceae)

wathiya*, *maanyarr (Y). The term ***maanyarr*** also was applied by some informants [(3), (7) : Y, B] to *Avicennia marina*; however no medicinal use was recorded for *A. marina*.

Use: Trunk or branches burned in a fire. Paste of ashes and water applied to sores, boils and ringworm [(2) : Y].

Brachychiton diversifolium (Sterculiaceae)

barlkparlk, *nhanhunngguwa* (Y); *burlkpurlk*, *burlgut*, *girrigitj* (D)

Use: Branches peeled and the wood crushed in water. Solution used as drops for sore eyes or as a wash to remove foreign particles [(2) : Y].

Buchanania arborescens (Anacardiaceae)

munydjutj (Y); the term *gatji'nganing* was recorded for *B. arborescens* (3), but with no medicinal use.

Use: Inner bark crushed or scraped into water and the infusion used for bathing sore eyes [(2) : Y].

Buchanania obovata (Anacardiaceae)

munydjutj, *dhurrpinda* (Y, B); *munydjutj*, *birrgi*, *baran.gurr* (D)

Use: Inner bark scraped into water and the mixture used for bathing sore eyes [(3) : Y]. Sapwood burnt and plugged in the cavity of a sore tooth. Leaves pounded and rubbed on the skin as a treatment for ringworm [(7) : D]. Wood-shavings packed into tooth for toothache (1). Material from this and *Calytrix exstipulata* mixed with red ant-bed (*gurndirr*) as a treatment for (? or protection from) mosquito and other insect bites [(7) : D]; details of the preparation not yet known.

Callitris intratropica (Cypressaceae)

lanapu (Y, B); *garn.gi* (D)

Use: Infusion of bark drunk for "sore belly" (? = diarrhoea). Ash from burnt stems rubbed on sore chest [(7) : D]. (See plate 5.)

Cansjera leptostachya (Opiliaceae)

dhuyuwurk (Y)

Use: Inner bark scraped into water and the mixture used for bathing sore eyes [(3), (2) : Y].

Capparis umbonata (Capparaceae)

burndjungu (D, B)

Use: Inner bark scraped into water, which is sometimes heated, and mixture washed over boils and cuts [(7) : D]. The infusion is drunk as a treatment for a sore throat and stomach pains (including diarrhoea) [(7) : D].

Carissa lanceolata (Apocynaceae)

djanyi (D)

Use: As a remedy for toothache [(7) : D].

Chrysopogon pallidus (Poaceae)

laawarr

Use: See under *Vigna vexillata.*

Cissus adnata (Vitidaceae)

yiiwirriny'-nganing (Y)

Use: Fruit crushed and placed on injuries from stingray barbs and cuts from oysters. Informants were a little unsure of this information [(3) : Y].

Clerodendron floribundum (Verbenaceae)

dutji, burulburul'-nganing (Y); *walpurrunggu'-ngining* (D)

Use: Either "inside bark" or crushed leaves soaked in water and the infusion rubbed on the body and sometimes drunk; used as a treatment for "sick stomach", coughs, colds and fever [(7) : D]. (See plates 1–3.)

Clerodendron sp. (Verbenaceae)

buwata'-nganing (Y)

Use: Leaves crushed in water and the patient is washed in the infusion; or given as a drink for head and backache, diarrhoea and vomiting [(2) : Y].

Crinum spp (Amaryllidaceae)

warrkarr (Y); *dhiitjpark, bakbakngarrak* (D)

Use: An onion-like root, the skins of which are used as dressings for serious wounds and infected sores. Wound or sore must be washed and dressed regularly [(2) : Y; (6), (7) : D].

Cycas media (Cycadaceae)

ngathu (B, Y); *ngathu, muthungay* (D)

Use: Wounds by iron or stone-head spear treated with the male flower stalk of *Cycas.* Male flower stalk split open and the soft centre obtained. This is cut into small pieces and placed in a paperbark basket, mixed with urine, warmed by the addition of hot stones and applied to the wound [(6), as *woragar,* Reeves (n.d.): *warraga*].

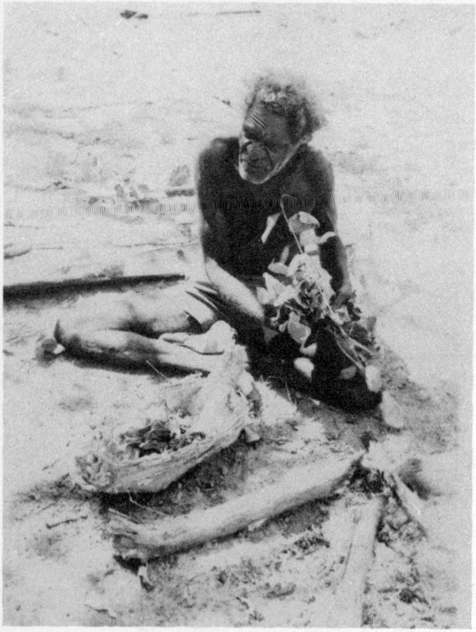

Steps in the preparation of *warl-purrunggu'-ngining* (*Clerodendron floribundum*), used by Dhulu-tarama at Donydji in April 1980 to treat the symptoms of influenza.

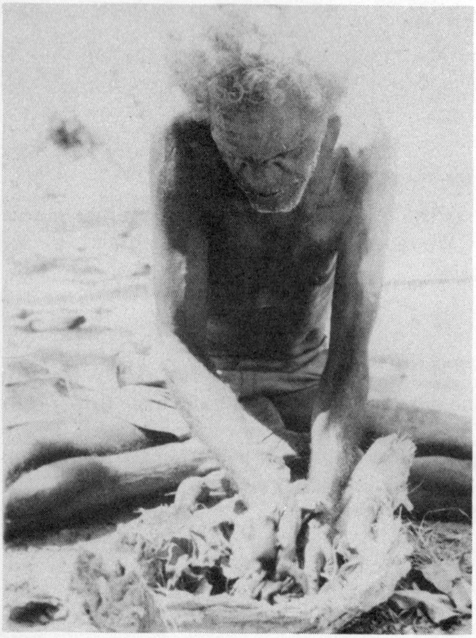

Leaves of *C. floribundum* are stripped and broken up into a paperbark container (*mungurr*), and hot water is poured over them.

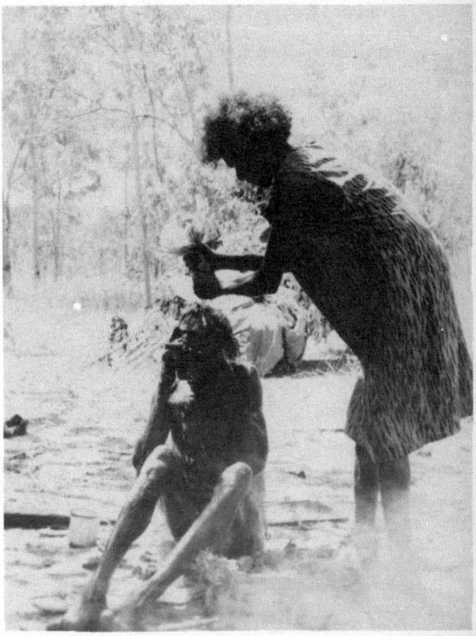

The infusion of *warlpurrunggu' ngining* is rubbed on the body and compressed over the head, chest and inner-thigh region, using a bark-wad (*mardarrbalk*). This is done in an effort to reduce fever and aches. On some occasions, the infusion is drunk.

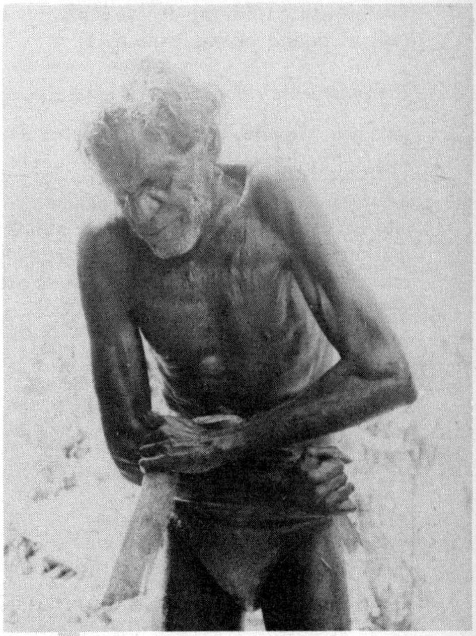

To conclude the treatment a strip (*gurla* : lit. "skin") of the inner bark of *garn.gi* (*Callitris intra-tropica*) is tied around the abdomen, to "make it feel better".

Cymbopogon spp (Poaceae)

gawurlurr-nganing (Y)

Use: Aromatic leaves of these grasses are rubbed into a ball and inhaled through the nose, to relieve colds [(3) : Y]. Infusion of leaves used as a liniment or drunk for influenzas, fevers, general aches and pains [(2), (6) : Y].

Dendrobium dicuphum (Orchidaceae)

djalkurrk (Y, D)

Use: Ends of the "stems" (pseudo-bulbs) are chewed and the mucilage dabbed on burns in cases where the skin has not been destroyed. Also applied to spear wounds [(6), (1)].

Denhamia obscura (Celastraceae)

dhurruringgitj (2), *durrurrur* (3) (Y); *garanggarang* (D)
Use: "Inside bark" is scraped off and placed in holes in the teeth to stop toothache, or a decoction of the wood is used for the same purpose [(3), (7) : Y, D; (2) : Y].

Eleocharis dulcis (Cyperaceae)

raakay (Y, B, D); *baaminyarr* (Y); *marpuy* (D)

Use: Moisture from the decaying plant is squeezed on burns and the rotting pulp is bound on the wound (1).

Erythrophleum chlorostachys (Caesalpiniaceae)

galanyin, maypiny, buutj, (Y); *maypiny* (D)

Use: Outer bark is placed on a fire and the patient sits over the smoke after a baby is born. She will not conceive a child again [(2) : Y]. Wood, leaves and bark used to smoke a person suffering from constipation (1). A preparation from the bark also is used to ease stomach pains [(7) : D]. Pulverized leaves sometimes are placed in the nostrils to reduce the discomfort of "diarrhoea" [(7) : D].

Eucalyptus miniata (Myrtaceae)

gungurru (Y, D)

Use: An infusion from inner bark and/or (?) leaves is used as a lotion for the treatment of swellings and as a tonic for diarrhoea [(7) : D].

Eucalyptus polycarpa (Myrtaceae)

warnduwa (Y); *dhumulu* (D)

Use: Kino (astringent gum) is dissolved in water and painted on ulcers and yaws. Treatment is repeated daily (6).

Eucalyptus tectifica (Myrtaceae)

warlan', *marrawalk* (inner bark preparation) (D)

Use: An infusion of the bark is drunk for "sore belly" and used externally for cuts and sores [(7) : D].

Eucalyptus tetradonta (Myrtaceae)

gardayka (Y, B, D); *ngardan* (D); *girrigirri* (inner bark, Y)

Use: Young coppice shoots (*dhunburutj*) are chewed for colds or crushed and placed on sores and cuts [(3) : Y]. An infusion of leaves or bark is drunk for aches and pains (particularly back pains) and for coughs [(7) : D; (6), (1)]. This infusion also is drunk to treat diarrhoea [(7) : D]. An infusion of inner bark is made in hot water and drunk to stop pain and bleeding after childbirth and to "bring on milk". Alternatively, the bark is put on a fire and the patient sits over the fire in the smoke [(2) : Y].

Ficus opposita, *F. scobina* (Moraceae)

muthi (Y, B, D)

Use: Inside bark scraped into water and the infusion used for treating sore eyes [(3) : Y]. This infusion is drunk to treat diarrhoea [(2) : D]. Leaves are crushed and steeped in water, then rubbed on the skin for muscular aches, influenzas and fevers (5).

Ficus racemosa (Moraceae)

muthi (Y)

Use: Scrapings of inner wood are placed in warm water, the patient drinks and is bathed in the infusion, to cure diarrhoea [(2) : Y].

Flagellaria indica (Flagellariaceae)

baaku (small form) (Y); *darwirr* (large form) (Y)

Use: Leaves are crushed and steeped in water and the infusion used as a linament for muscular aches, influenzas and fevers; also taken internally [(2), Y; (6)]. The young shoots are chewed to prevent toothache [(D) and (Y), 1979].

Gardenia megasperma (Rubiaceae)

burrparndala (D)

Use: Fruit is used to treat toothache [(7) : D].

Grewia retusifolia (Tiliaceae)

murrnyi or *murrtjumun* (Y); *murrnyi* (B, D)

Use: Leaves pounded, placed in water and put on wounds and cuts. The roots are used to soften boils: the inner bark of the roots is scraped off, beaten between stones, soaked in water and placed on the boil until it is soft and the pus can be removed [(3), (7) : Y, B; (4)]. An infusion of the roots also may be drunk to cure diarrhoea (4), or for "the heart" [(7) : D].

Helicteres cana (Sterculiaceae)

maari'mirringu murrtjumun (Y)

Use. Inner bark of the roots is scraped off, beaten between stones, soaked in water and placed on boils to soften them [(3) : Y]. The plant is named from ***murrtjumun*** (*Grewia retusifolia*; q.v.), which it resembles, both in appearance and use.

Hibiscus tiliaceus (Malvaceae)

marlwan, yaarl, mapandurr (Y)

Use: Inner "wood" scraped into water and put on sores as a "drawer" for boils [(2) : Y]. The freshly stripped bark is used to bind wounds [(3) : Y]. Internal use for deep wounds was reported by (1).

Hypoestes floribunda (Acanthaceae)

garlpu-nganing (Y)

Use: Whole plant was mashed up and inhaled for colds, or used on sores [(3) : Y].

Ipomoea pescaprae (L.) Sweet (Convolvulaceae)

ruuwu (Y)

Use: Heated leaves of this species are applied to catfish, stingray and post-circumcision wounds. In the case of catfish and stingray wounds, crushed cockroaches (***buurduk***) are added [(2) : Y, (6)].

Litsea ?glutinosa (Lauraceae)

butjiri-nganing (Y); also applied to *Polyalthia holtzeana* (q.v.)

Use: Leaves are used as a "rubbing medicine" or liniment on sore muscles [(3) : Y]. An infusion of the leaves in water is drunk to cure vomiting [(7) : D].

Melaleuca acacioides (Myrtaceae)

gurlu'kurlun' (D)

Use: An infusion of the leaves is drunk for "sore belly" [(7), (3) : D].

Melaleuca cajuputi (Myrtaceae)

nhaambarra, barrtjiray (Y); ***djiirri*** (D)

Use: Leaves are crushed and inhaled to relieve colds. An infusion of leaves with *malak* (green ants) is drunk for colds, and without *malak* for "bad liver". The leaves are heated on the fire and rubbed on the head and arms to relieve headaches [(3) (7) : Y, D].

Melaleuca leucadendron (Myrtaceae)

dhurlgu (Y, D); *wuurlk* (Y)

Use: Inner bark is mashed and put in warm water; the patient drinks this and is bathed with the infusion. Treats headaches, backaches and colds [(2) : Y]. Bark used for bandages [(7) : D]. The term *wuurlk* also was applied to an unusual form of *M. dealbata* by one informant (3); no medical use for *dealbata* was recorded, however.

Melaleuca viridiflora (Myrtaceae)

nhaambarra (Y)

Use: Young leaves are crushed in hot water and the patient is bathed in the infusion; used to treat colds and influenza [(2) : Y].

Morinda citrifolia (Rubiaceae)

burukpili (Y, B); *djinbirrk* (D); *gurninyi* [(6), Milingimbi]

Use: Green fruit is crushed and eaten to cure diarrhoea [(3), (7) : Y, B; (6)]. Leaves are crushed, placed in water and the infusion used as a liniment for influenza, fevers and general aches and pains. (1) states that an infusion also was drunk for diarrhoea.

Owenia vernicosa (Meliaceae)

djin.giritj, ngarna' (D)

Use: Heated leaves are used in the treatment of sore eyes and headache [(7) : D].

Pandanus spiralis R.Br. (Pandanaceae) *P. whitei* Martelli [according to (4)]

gun.ga (Y); *gun.ga, gundjak* (D)

Use: Pith of the tree is crushed and the white liquid that is expressed is mixed with water and applied to wounds or sores. The mixture also is gargled for toothache, mouth and throat sores [(2) : Y]. Pith of the stem is mixed with urine and applied hot to ulcers, yaws and similar diseases [(3) : Y, (6)].

Persoonia falcata (Proteaceae)

dan.gapa, barlwa (Y, B); *dhan.gapa', dhagirritj* (D)

Use: Inner bark soaked in water and the infusion used for sore eyes [Warner, 1958; (5)]. Fruit also is used for the eyes [(3), (7) : D].

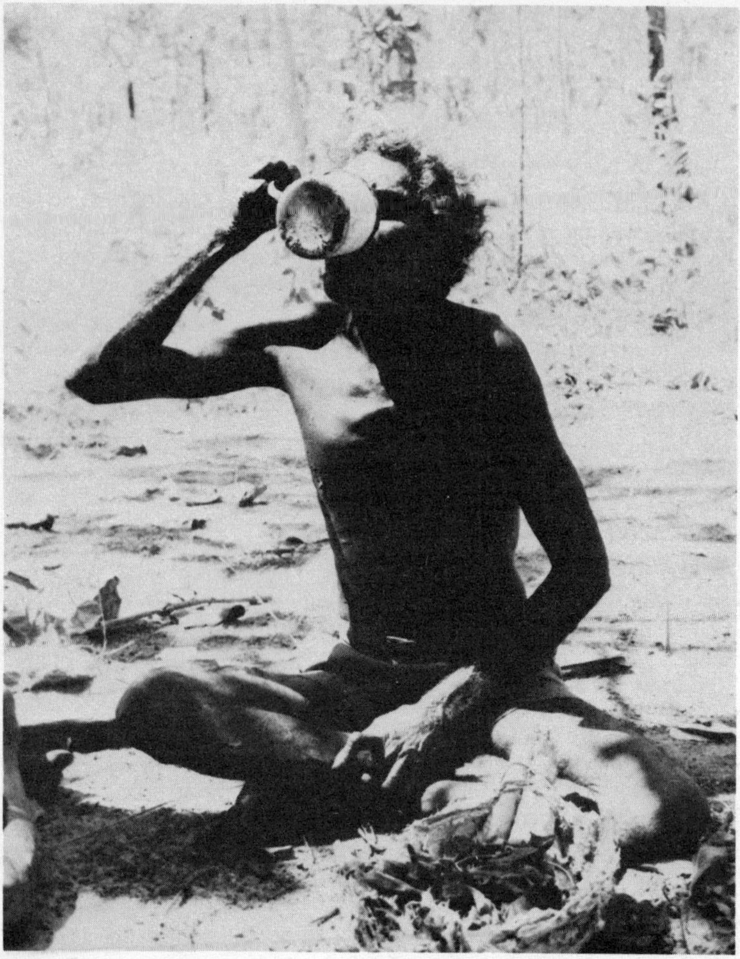

Lightly charred *mangarnmangarn* (a shelf fungus, *Phellinus rimosus*) is scraped into water and drunk, to relieve coughing and when "no good inside, near heart".

Phellinus spp

dakul'-nganing (*P. robustus* [Korst.] Bourd and Galz); ***bulungun*** (Y); ***mangarnmangarn*** (D) (*P. rimosus* [Berk] Pil.)

Use: For "sores in the throat". The fungus is chopped from the tree and placed on a fire and the patient inhales the smoke. Lightly charred ***bulungun*** is scraped into the water and the patient drinks the infusion [(2) : Y]. Prepared in this way, it also is used in the treatment of coughs and "bad chest", and when feverish [(7) : D]. (See plate 4.)

Planchonia careya (Barringtoniaceae)

dhanggi, djalalu, murrbunbun (Y, B, D)

Use: Bark used as a hot poultice on sores from granuloma and yaws, and on spear wounds [Warner, 1958 (5)]. As for *djin.giritj* (*Owenia vernicosa*), heated leaves are placed on the forehead to ease/cure headache, especially when "troubled" (*wargugu*) [(7) : D].

Polyalthia holtzeana (Anonaceae)

butjiri-nganing (Y); also applied to *Litsea ?glutinosa* (q.v.)

Use: Leaves are crushed in water and the patient is washed in the infusion to treat general illnesses. Infusion also is dropped into the ear to treat sore ears [(2) : Y].

Premna acuminata (Verbenaceae)

wakmanggarr (Y) (also "roughly" *dutji*); *dhurruman'* (D)

Use: Wood and bark are used to splint broken bones [(7) : D].

Rhizophora stylosa (Rhizophoraceae)

walmu (Y)

Use: Inner bark is scraped into water and the infusion used to treat ulcers and yaws (6). Webb (1933) uses the term *barnggor* (black mangrove), of Macassan origin, cf. Bahasa Indonesia *bakau.*

Sarcocephalus coadunata (Roxb. ex J. E. Sm.) Druce (Rubiaceae)

burukpili (Y)

Use: Pounded fruit and seeds are placed in water and drunk for headaches, vomiting, diarrhoea, colds and pains in the stomach [(2) : Y].

Scaevola taccada (Gaertn.) Roxb. (Goodeniaceae)

warnarrambarr (Y, B)

Use: Ripe fruit is heated in hot sand and the juice is squeezed into sore eyes [(3) : Y].

Smilax australis (Smilacaceae)

dapu (Y, D)

Use: An extract from this plant used to treat sore eyes [(7) : D].

Sterculia quadrifida (Sterculiaceae)

barlkparlk (Y, B, D); *burlkpurlk* (D)

Use: Inner bark scraped into water or breast milk and the infusion used on sore eyes [(3), (7) : Y, B; (5)].

Syzygium suborbiculare (Benth.) Hartley et Perry (Myrtaceae)

larrarni (Y, B); *burrumu* (D)

Use: Young leaves are soaked in water and the infusion is drunk for diarrhoea [(7) :]. An infusion of the bark and leaves in water is used to bathe sores. Pulp of the cooked fruit is put in sore ears [(7) : D].

Terminalia carpentariae (Combretaceae)

mamarnbu (Y, B); *mapurdumun'*, *ngaraminy* (D)

Use: Red sap from inner bark is scraped off, pounded and rubbed on swollen feet as a liniment [(3) : Y]. (6) mentions this species under the name *balparangan*.

Terminalia ferdinandiana Exell (Combretaceae)

mamarnbu, *mupan* (Y)

Use: Slices of the inner bark are pounded between stones and mixed in cold water. The patient is bathed in the infusion, which remains on the skin as a sticky paste. Used to treat sores (including leprous patches), backaches and sore feet [(2) : Y].

Tinospora smilacina (Menispermaceae)

burrpuy (Y)

Use: Leaves used in a poultice for stingray wounds; the leaves are heated in the hot ashes of a fire and cockroaches (*buurduk*) are crushed and added to the hot leaves. The mixture is then placed on the wound and bound with the bark of the *Tinospora* vine [(3), Y; (6)].

Trema aspera (Ulmaceae)

buwalawal (Y)

Use: Leaves are pounded, placed in water and plastered on spear wounds. Informant stated that it was used "*ngaathilingu*", i.e. in former times, not at present [(3) : Y].

Vigna vexillata (Fabaceae)

gulparung, *yukuwa* (Y, B, D); *bunbun* (D)

Use: T. Webb (1933) states that *dirrbuk*, a small carrot-like root, was pounded between stones with *lauwarr*, a kind of grass, and inserted into the abdominal cavity when the intestines were put back into the cavity after a severe abdominal wound. Reeves (n.d.) records the term *dhirmbuk* for V. vexillata, a species with an edible tap-root. Reeve's *lawarr* (*Chrysopogon pallidus*) is almost certainly the grass *lauwarr* of Webb.

Xylocarpus australasicus, Ridl. (Meliaceae)

gukawu (Y)

Use: Inner bark is crushed in water and drunk for "any illness" [(2) : Y].

ALPHABETIC INDEX OF YOLNGU NAMES

Yolngu Term	Plant Species
baaku	*Flagellaria indica*
baaminyarr	*Eleocharis dulcis*
bakbakngarrak	*Crinum* spp
balparangan	*Terminalia carpentariae*
baran.gurr	*Buchanania obovata*
barlkparlk	*Sterculia quadrifida, Brachychiton diversifolium*
barlwa	*Persoonia falcata*
barrtjiray	*Melaleuca cajuputi*
birrgi	*Buchanania obovata*
bulungun	*Phellinus rimosus*
bunbun	*Vigna vexillata*
burlgut	*Brachychiton diversifolium*
burlkpurlk	*Sterculia quadrifida, Brachychiton diversifolium*
burndjungu	*Capparis umbonata*
burrparndala	*Gardenia megasperma*
burrpuy	*Tinospora smilacina*
burrumu	*Syzygium suborbiculare*
burukpili	*Morinda citrifolia* (3), *Sarcocephalus coadunata* (2)
burulburul'-nganing	*Clerodendron floribundum*
butjiri-nganing	*Litsea ?glutinosa* (3), *Polyalthia holtzeana* (2)
buutj	*Erythrophleum chlorostachys*
buwalawal	*Trema aspera*
buwata'-nganing	*Clerodendron* sp.
dakul'-nganing	*Phellinus robustus*
dan.gapa	*Persoonia falcata*
dapu	*Smilax australis*
darwirr	*Flagellaria indica*
dhagirritj	*Persoonia falcata*
dhan.gapa'	*Persoonia falcata*
dhanggi	*Planchonia careya*
dhiitjpark	*Crinum* spp
dhirmbuk	*Vigna vexillata*
dhumulu	*Eucalyptus polycarpa*
dhurlgu	*Melaleuca leucadendron*
dhurrpinda	*Buchanania obovata*
dhurruman'	*Premna acuminata*
dhurruringgitj	*Denhamia obscura*

dhuyuwurk	*Cansjera leptostachya*
djalala	*Planchonia careya*
djalkurrk	*Dendrobium dicuphum*
djanyi	*Carissa lanceolata*
djiirri	*Melaleuca cajuputi*
djinbirrk	*Morinda citrifolia*
djin.giritj	*Owenia vernicosa*
durrurrur	*Denhamia obscura*
dutji	*Clerodendron floribundum*
galanyin	*Erythrophleum chlorostachys*
garanggarang	*Denhamia obscura*
gardayka	*Eucalyptus tetradonta*
garlpu-nganing	*Hypoestes floribunda*
garn.gi	*Callitris intratropica*
gawurlurr-nganing	*Cymbopogon* spp
girrigirri	*Eucalyptus tetradonta* (inner bark)
girrigitj	*Brachychiton diversifolium*
gukawu	*Xylocarpus australasicus*
gulparung	*Vigna vexillata*
gundjak	*Pandanus spiralis*
gun.ga	*Pandanus spiralis, P. whitei*
gungurru	*Eucalyptus miniata*
gurlu'kurlun	*Melaleuca acacioides*
gurninyi	*Morinda citrifolia*
laawarr	*Chrysopogon pallidus*
lanapu	*Callitris intratropica* (endemic)
larrarni	*Syzygium suborbiculare*
maanyarr	*Alphitonia petrei* (2), *Avicennia marina* (3)
maari'mirringu murrtjumun	*Helicteres cana*
mamarnbu	*Terminalia carpentariae* (3), *T. ferdinandiana* (2)
mangarnmangarn	*Phellinus rimosus*
mapandurr	*Hibiscus tiliaceus*
mapurdumun'	*Terminalia carpentariae*
marlwan	*Hibiscus tiliaceus*
marpuy	*Eleocharis dulcis*
marrawalk	*Eucalyptus tectifica* (inner bark)
maypiny	*Erythrophleum chlorostachys*
munydjutj	*Buchanania obovata* (3) (7); *B. arborescens* (2)
mupan	*Terminalia ferdinandiana*
murrbunbun	*Planchonia careya*
murrnyi	*Grewia retusifolia*

murrtjumun	*Grewia retusifolia*
muthi	*Ficus opposita, F. scobina* (3), *F. racemosa* (2)
muthungay	*Cycas media*
ngaraminy	*Terminalia carpentariae*
ngardan	*Eucalyptus tetradonta*
ngarnạ'	*Owenia vernicosa*
ngathu	*Cycas media*
nhaambarra	*Melaleuca cajuputi* (3); *M. viridiflora* (2)
nhanhungguwa	*Brachychiton diversifolium*
raakay	*Eleocharis dulcis*
ruuwu	*Ipomoea pescaprae*
wakmanggarr	*Premna acuminata*
walmu	*Rhizophora stylosa*
walpurrunggu'-ngining	*Clerodendron floribundum*
warlan'	*Eucalyptus tectifica*
warnarrambarr	*Scaevola taccada*
warnduwa	*Eucalyptus polycarpa*
warraga (woragar)	*Cycas media*
warrkarr	*Crinum* spp
wathiya	*Alphitonia petrei*
wuurlk	*Melaleuca leucadendron* (2), *M. dealbata* (3)
yaarl	*Hibiscus tiliaceus*
yiiwirriny'-nganing	*Cissus adnata*
yukuwa	*Vigna vexillata*

CLASSIFICATION OF MEDICINAL PLANTS IN TERMS OF USE (AFTER L. J. WEBB, 1969)

External

BODY PAINS AND GENERAL MALAISE

Callitris intratropica
Clerodendron floribundum
Clerodendron sp.
Cymbopogon spp
Erythrophleum chlorostachys
Ficus opposita
Ficus scobina
Flagellaria indica
Litsea ?glutinosa
Melaleuca cajuputi
Melaleuca leucadendron
Morinda citrifolia
Owenia vernicosa
Planchonia careya
Polyalthia holtzeana
Terminalia carpentariae
Terminalia ferdinandiana

COUGHS, COLDS AND LUNG COMPLAINTS

Clerodendron floribundum
Clerodendron sp.
Cymbopogon spp
Eucalyptus tetradonta
Ficus opposita
Ficus scobina
Flagellaria indica
Melaleuca leucadendron
Melaleuca viridiflora
Morinda citrifolia

EYES

Brachychiton diversifolium
Buchanania arborescens
Buchanania obovata
Cansjera leptostachya
Ficus opposita
Ficus scobina
Owenia vernicosa
Persoonia falcata
Scaevola taccada
Smilax australis
Sterculia quadrifida

TEETH

Buchanania arborescens
Buchanania obovata
Carissa lanceolata
Denhamia obscura
Flagellaria indica
Gardenia megasperma
Pandanus spiralis
Pandanus whitei

SKIN LESIONS AND WOUNDS

Alphitonia petrei
Avicennia marina
Buchanania arborescens
Buchanania obovata
Capparis umbonata
Cissus adnata (?)
Crinum spp
Cycas media
Dendrobium dicuphum
Eleocharis dulcis
Eucalyptus miniata
Eucalyptus polycarpa
Eucalyptus tectifica
Eucalyptus tetradonta
Grewia retusifolia
Helicteres cana
Hibiscus tiliaceus
Hypoestes floribunda
Ipomoea pescaprae
Pandanus spiralis
Pandanus whitei
Phellinus rimosus
Phellinus robustus
Planchonia careya
Rhizophora stylosa
Syzygium suborbiculare
Terminalia ferdinandiana
Trema aspera

SKIN BITES AND STINGS

Buchanania obovata
Calytrix exstipulata
Cissus adnata
Ipomoea pescaprae
Tinospora smilacina

MISCELLANEOUS

Hibiscus tiliaceus (bandages)
Melaleuca leucadendron (bandages)
Polyalthia holtzeana
Premna acuminata (splints for broken bones)
Tinospora vine (bandages)

Internal

BODY PAINS AND GENERAL MALAISE

Callitris intratropica
Clerodendron floribundum
Clerodendron sp.
Cymbopogon spp
Eucalyptus tetradonta
Flagellaria indica
Grewia retusifolia
Melaleuca leucadendron
Phellinus rimosus
Sarcocephalus coadunata

COUGHS, COLDS AND LUNG COMPLAINTS

Cansjera leptostachya
Capparis umbonata
Clerodendron floribundum
Cymbopogon spp
Eucalyptus tetradonta
Flagellaria indica
Hypoestes floribunda
Melaleuca cajuputi
Melaleuca leucadendron
Melaleuca viridiflora
Pandanus spiralis
Pandanus whitei
Phellinus rimosus
Phellinus robustus
Sarcocephalus coadunata

GASTRO-INTESTINAL

Callitris intratropica
Capparis umbonata
Clerodendron floribundum
Clerodendron sp.
Cymbopogon spp
Erythrophleum chlorostachys
Eucalyptus miniata
Eucalyptus tectifica
Eucalyptus tetradonta
Ficus opposita
Ficus racemosa
Ficus scobina
Grewia retusifolia
Litsea ?glutinosa
Melaleuca acacioides
Melaleuca cajuputi
Morinda citrifolia
Sarcocephalus coadunata
Syzygium suborbiculare

EARS

Polyalthia holtzeana
Syzygium suborbiculare

WOUNDS (deep, abdominal)

Chrysopogon pallidus
Hibiscus tiliaceus
Vigna vexillata

MISCELLANEOUS

Xylocarpus australasicus

NOTES

1 The transcription of Yolngu terms follows the Australian Institute of Aboriginal Studies convention for the representation of tribal and language names, with the following qualifications:
(a) The retroflexed rhotic is represented by *r* and the trilled rhotic by *rr*.
(b) Word initial retroflexed stops are unmarked; medial and final retroflexed stops are represented by the digraphs *rd*, *rn*, etc.
(c) The velar nasal is transcribed by *ng*, the alveolar nasal plus nasal stop by *n.g*.
(d) Long vowels are represented by doubling the letter.

[2] There are some apparent discrepancies in the data listed in the appendix, particularly in the application of Yolngu terms to certain taxa, e.g. the various *Melaleuca* species. In this case, four closely related species are involved, which occur in the field in a great variety of growth forms; the distinction between these species was elucidated only relatively recently (Blake, 1968). The Yolngu classification may operate on the basis of features regarded as relatively unimportant by taxonomists, e.g. size, growth form, bark thickness, etc. Other apparent inconsistencies may be due to misunderstandings or misidentifications by either the investigator or the informants. It should be noted that often several plant species with the same general appearance or use are grouped under one term, resulting in a degree of confusion for the investigator. Moreover, different terms for the same plant may arise through dialect differences or from the practice of employing a variety of alternative names for some species. For instance, a man with a name which sounded like *munydjutj* died in 1981 and, since then, the tree has been called only *dhurrpinda.* (The names of the recently deceased and similar sounding words may not be said.) The precise usage of a shared name also may vary from dialect to dialect or from group to group. In view of these points, the degree of consistency between the two sets of results (Reid v. Scarlett/White) is perhaps surprising.

REFERENCES

Bell, D., 1978. "Ritual and Reality: Aboriginal Women's Health in a Desert Community" (Paper read at the Australian Anthropological Society Conference, University of Sydney, 31 August 1978), p. 4.

Berndt, R. M., 1955. " 'Murngin' (Wulamba) Social Organization", *American Anthropology* 57 : 84–106.

——, 1965. "Marriage and the Family in North-eastern Arnhem Land", in *Comparative Family Systems*, ed. M. F. Nimkoff (Boston : Houghton Mifflin), pp. 77–104.

——, and Berndt, C. H., 1954. *Arnhem Land, Its History and Its People* (Melbourne : Cheshire).

—— and ——, 1970. *Man, Land and Myth in North Australia: The Gunwinggu People* (Sydney : Ure Smith).

Black, R. H., 1972. *Malaria in Australia* (Canberra : Australian Government Publishing Service).

Blake, S. T., 1968. "A Revision of *Melaleuca leucadendron* and Its Allies", *Contributions Queensland He barium*, no. 1 : 1–114.

Burkill, I. H., 1966. *A Dictionary of the Economic Products of the Malay Peninsula* (Kuala Lumpur : Art Printing Works).

Cawte, J. E., 1974. *Medicine is the Law* (Honolulu : University Press of Hawaii).

Chaseling, W. S., 1957. *Yulengor: Nomads of Arnhem Land* (London : Epworth Press).

Chippendale, G. M., 1971. "Check List of Northern Territory Plants", *Proceedings Linnean Society of New South Wales* 96 : 207–67.

Cook, C. E., 1970. Notable Changes in the Incidence of Disease in Northern Territory Aborigines", in *Diprotodon to Detribalization*, ed. A. R. Pilling and R. A. Waterman (Michigan : Michigan State University Press) pp. 116–30.

Djaypila and Yalwidika, 1979. "Medicinal Plants on Elcho Island", *Aboriginal Health Worker* 3 : 50–56.
Doherty, R. L., 1973. "The Health Status of Aboriginal Communities in Cape York Peninsula", in *The Human Biology of Aborigines in Cape York*, ed. R. L. Kirk (Canberra : Australian Institute of Aboriginal Studies), pp. 37–48.
Dunlop, C. R., Latz, P. K., and Maconochie, J. R., 1976. "A Botanical Survey of Elcho Island, July 1975", *Northern Territory Botany Bulletin* 1 : 1–61.
Eastwell, H. D., 1973. "The Traditional Healer in Modern Arnhem Land", *Medical Journal of Australia* 2 : 1011–17..
Elkin, A. P., 1977. *Aboriginal Men of High Degree* (St Lucia : University of Queensland Press, 2nd edn); first published 1945.
Elphinstone, J. J., 1971. "The Health of Australian Aborigines with no Previous Association with Europeans", *Medical Journal of Australia* 2 : 293.
Golson, J., 1971. "Australian Aboriginal Food Plants: Some Ecological and Culture-historical Implications", in *Aboriginal Man and Environment in Australia*, ed. D. J. Mulvaney and J. Golson (Canberra : Australian National University Press), pp. 196–238.
Heath, J., 1978. *Ngandi Grammar, Texts and Dictionary* (Canberra : Australian Institute of Aboriginal Studies. New Jersey : Humanities Press).
———, 1980. *Basic Materials in Ritharngu: Grammar, Texts and Dictionary*, Pacific Linguistics Series B. no. 62, ed. S. A. Wurm (Canberra : Australian National University, School of Pacific Studies, Department of Linguistics).
Kirke, D. K., 1974. "The Traditionally Oriented Community", in *Better Health for Aborigines?*, ed. B. S. Hetzel, M. Dobbin, L. Lippman and E. Eggleston (St Lucia : University of Queensland Press), pp. 81–87.
Levitt, D., 1979. "Unwritten Pharmacopoeia", *Hemisphere* 23 : 244–49.
———, 1981. *Plants and People: Aboriginal Uses of Plants in Groote Eylandt* (Canberra : Australian Institute of Aboriginal Studies).
McArthur, M., 1960. "Report of the Nutrition Unit. 6. Food Consumption and Dietary Levels of Groups of Aborigines Living on Naturally Occurring Foods", in *Records of the American-Australian Scientific Expedition to Arnhem Land*, vol. 2, *Anthropology and Nutrition*, ed. C. P. Mountford (Melbourne : Melbourne University Press), pp. 90–135.
MacKnight, C. C., 1972. "Macassans and Aborigines", *Oceania* 42 : 283–321.
Meehan, B., 1977. "Hunters by the Seashore", *Journal of Human Evolution* 6, no. 4 : 363–70.
Moodie, P. M., 1973. *Aboriginal Health*, Aborigines in Australian Society 9 (Canberra : Australian National University Press).
Morphy, H., 1978. "Rights in Paintings and Rights in Women: A Consideration of Some of the Basic Problems Posed by the Asymmetry of the '*Murngin* System' ", *Mankind* 11 : 208–19.
Mountford, C. P. (ed.), 1956. *Records of the American–Australian Scientific Expedition to Arnhem Land*, vol. 1, *Art, Myth and Symbolism* (Melbourne : Melbourne University Press).
Mulvaney, D. J., 1969. *The Prehistory of Australia* (London : Thames and Hudson).

Neel, J. and V., 1977. "Health and Disease in Unacculturated Amerindian Populations", in *Health and Disease in Tribal Societies*, Ciba Foundation Symposium 49 (Amsterdam : Elsevier, Excerpta Medica), pp. 155–68.

Powell, J. M., 1976. "Ethnobotany", in *New Guinea Vegetation*, ed. K. Paijmans (Canberra : Australian National University Press), pp. 106–99.

Reeves, H. (n.d.). Unpublished, untitled ms. (Canberra : Australian Institute of Aboriginal Studies library).

Reid, J. C., 1978a. "The Role of the *Marrnggitj* in Contemporary Health Care", *Oceania* 49, no. 2 : 96–109.

——, Forthcoming. *Spirits, Sorcerers, and Strangers* (Canberra: Australia National University Press).

——, and Mununggurr, D., 1977. "We are Losing Our Brothers: Sorcery and Alcohol in an Aboriginal Community", *Medical Journal of Australia* (Special Supplement) 2 : 1–5.

Schebeck, B., n.d. "Dialect and Social Groupings in North-east Arnhem Land", unpublished ms. (Canberra : Australian Institute of Aboriginal Studies).

——, 1970. In *A Revised Linguistic Survey of Australia*, ed. W. J. and L. F. Oates (Canberra : Australian Institute of Aboriginal Studies), pp. 225–26.

Specht, R. L., 1958. "The Climate, Geology, Soils and Plant Ecology of the Northern Portion of Arnhem Land", in *Records of the American-Australian Scientific Expedition to Arnhem Land*, vol. 3, *Botany and Plant Ecology*, ed. R. L. Specht and C. P. Mountford (Melbourne : Melbourne University Press), pp. 333–413.

Straatmans, W., 1967. "Ethnobotany of New Guinea in its Ecological Perspective", *Journal d'agriculture tropicale et de botanique appliquée* 14 : 1–20.

——, n.d. "An Ethno-botanical Check List of New Guinea", unpublished ms. (Canberra : New Guinea Research Unit, Australian National University).

Taylor, J. C., 1977. "A Pre-contact Aboriginal Medical System on Cape York Peninsula", *Journal of Human Evolution* 6 : 419–32.

Thomson, D. F., 1961. "Marrngitmirri and Kalka — Medicineman and Sorcerer — in Arnhem Land", *Man* 61 : 97–102.

Tindale, N. B., 1925. "Natives of Groote Eylandt and of the West Coast of the Gulf of Carpentaria", *Records South Australian Museum* 2, no. 1 : 61–102; 3, no. 2 : 103–34.

Truswell, A. S., 1977. "Diet and Nutrition of Hunter-gatherers", in *Health and Disease in Tribal Societies*, Ciba Foundation Symposium 49 (Amsterdam : Elsevier, Excerpta Medica), pp. 213–21.

Warner, W. L., 1958. *A Black Civilization: A Social Study of an Australian Tribe* (New York : Harper and Row; first published 1937; Torchbook edn, 1964).

Webb, L. J., 1969. "The Use of Plant Medicines and Poisons by Australian Aborigines", *Mankind* 7 : 137–46.

——, 1973. " 'Eat, Die and Learn' — The Botany of the Australian Aborigines", *Australian Natural History* 7, no. 9 : 290–95.

Webb, T. T., 1933. "Aboriginal Medical Practice in East Arnhem Land", *Oceania* 4 : 91–98.

——, 1936. "The Making of a Marrngit", *Oceania* 6 : 336–41.

White, I. M., 1977. "Pitfalls to Avoid: The Australian Experience", in *Health and Disease in Tribal Societies*, Ciba Foundation Symposium 49 (Amsterdam : Elsevier, Excerpta Medica), pp. 269–301.

White, N. G., 1976. "A Preliminary Account of the Correspondence among Genetic, Linguistic, Social and Topographic Divisions in Arnhem Land, Australia", *Mankind* 10 : 240–47.

——, 1978. A Human Ecology Research Project in the Arnhem Land Region: An Outline", Australian Institute of Aboriginal Studies *Newsletter* (new series), no. 9 : 39–52.

——, 1979. "Tribes, Genes and Habitats: Genetic Diversity among Aboriginal Populations in the Northern Territory of Australia" (Ph.D. thesis, La Trobe University).

Wilson, W., 1953. "A Dietary Survey of Aborigines in the Northern Territory", *Medical Journal of Australia* 2, no. 16 : 599–605.

Wise, P. H., Edwards, F. M., Craig, R. J. Evans, B., Murchland, J. M., Sutherland, B., and Thomas, D. W., 1976. "Diabetes and Associated Variables in the South Australian Aboriginal", *Australia New Zealand Journal of Medicine* 6 : 191–96.

Part Three

Medical Strategies in Change

Studies of the impact of social change on the indigenous medical systems of many societies have shown that, while the people often adapt their traditional strategies for dealing with illness to take advantage of Western medicine, they retain their own perspectives on sickness, death and curing, and continue to explain these phenomena in traditional ways. Research in Aboriginal communities has indicated a similar pattern. The Yolngu of Arnhem Land, for instance, now look to the introduced medical service for treatment of the majority of their illnesses, but continue to draw on their own medical theory to explain the causes of these illnesses. Although their theory of illness originated in a social environment quite unlike that of today, it remains very relevant to the Yolngu for several reasons: unlike Western medicine, it explains illness at several different levels (what, how and why); it is an integral part of the social and religious life of the community; it can encompass change; and it logically explains the relationship between contemporary social crises and illness. In a way Western concepts of causality cannot, the indigenous theory orders experience, reinforces social values, explains misfortune and gives a sense of mastery over what would otherwise appear a capricious and unpredictable cosmos.[1]

The two concluding chapters of this book are analyses of the theoretical and practical adaptations that two other Aboriginal communities have made to the reduced and changing circumstances in which they find themselves. These studies show that the Aboriginal people of central Australia, like the Yolngu, have seen fit to incorporate useful elements of Western medicine into their medical repertoire, but still conceptualize and cope with sickness in a uniquely Aboriginal way.

Diane Bell's chapter, "Women's Changing Role in Health Maintenance in a Central Australian Community", focuses on the Aboriginal women of Warrabri. Bell shows that these women are not extras in the play of life and death. They are protagonists. In the past, their role in maintaining health and harmony was critical to the survival of their society. Today they live in a radically altered world, where they are struggling to maintain their role in health maintenance. In part, the women are doing this through ritual, but their ritual modes of expressing concern for health are changing. Bell argues that, although women living on this and other large government settlements may have more opportunities to stage rituals, the loss of land over which they foraged, and from which they derived their identity, has deprived them of their power-base. In the past, the women of Warrabri were independent and autonomous; today they are dependent. Nevertheless, they continue to assert their role as nurturers of people and country. Part of this role is to confront and attempt to remedy the social disharmonies that are, in their view, making their people sick.

Myrna Tonkinson's study, "The *Mabarn* and the Hospital: The Selection of Treatment in a Remote Aboriginal Community", delineates the rich set of traditional resources available to people of Jigalong in the Western desert when they are sick. She focuses particularly on the role of the *mabarn*, or Aboriginal doctor, in healing and health maintenance, and compares the use of traditional curing methods with those provided by Western medical services.

Tonkinson's research shows that the people of Jigalong regard both Aboriginal and Western modes of treatment as effective and, depending on the type of illness, call upon either or both with little apparent conflict. Research all over the world has revealed a similar pattern. People are pragmatic in their search for a cure for an illness: they will utilize whatever resources are accessible to them. It is not necessarily the case, though, that changes in practice reflect changes in belief. In Aboriginal communities, a coherent body of medical thought shapes the interpretations of misfortune among young and old. The indigenous medical system, as Tonkinson so clearly shows, remains a powerful force, influencing the community's reaction to sickness and, as Bell shows, its view of social processes.

NOTES

[1] J. C. Reid, "Change in the Indigenous Medical System of an Aboriginal Community", *Australian Institute of Aboriginal Studies Newsletter* (1978): 9 : 61–72.

9
Women's Changing Role in Health Maintenance in a Central Australian Community

Diane Bell

INTRODUCTION

A century of European colonization of Central Australia has wrought dramatic changes in the lives of desert Aborigines whose traditional country is now alienated by mining, pastoral and industrial-urban interests. The ensuing shift from a semi-nomadic lifestyle of small bands of hunter-gatherers to the sedentary lifestyle of large government settlements, missions, cattle-stations and towns has created new tensions and intensified old conflicts. In the face of dislocation, dispossession and violence, Central Australian Aborigines have maintained a distinctively Aboriginal lifestyle which continues to have meaning for them in their rapidly changing situation. The impact of the changes of the last century on the health of Aborigines is of concern to both the people themselves and to the government agencies delivering health services and care. In this chapter, some of the changes and continuities in the domain of health maintenance as perceived by the Kaititj women of Warrabri, a government settlement some 375 kilometres north of Alice Springs in the Northern Territory, are explored.

Women's perceptions of the changes in their lives, it is argued, are given ritual expression in women's ceremonies, many of which directly or indirectly concern the health and well-being of members of their society. In the past, many women's ceremonies centred on crises of life — birth, death, menarche — and the health of the small, intimately related band in which people lived most of the year. Today women's ceremonies centre upon resolution of conflict within the larger, more diffuse groups of people with whom they now live on settlements. Women have continued to assert their nurturing role, but in the past the range of expression and constraints on this role were of a different order from today. As their circumstances have changed, women have responded by turning to and emphasizing different aspects of their ritual repertoire. The shifts in focus, structure and content of women's ceremonies are a key to understanding women's changing role in the domain of health, as they perceive it.

Scant attention has been paid to women's attitudes concerning the domain of health and to their role in maintaining the health of their families and the communities in which they live. There are, it is suggested, two interrelated reasons for this neglect. The broad-ranging nature of the indigenous concepts of health and disease in Aboriginal Australia have been hazily understood by many anthropologists and medical personnel, who have focused on the spectacular role of the traditional healer.[1] This has been coupled with an even more profound misunderstanding of the usurpation and erosion of women's autonomous role. During the past century of contact, European institutions such as schools, hospitals and welfare agencies have severely undermined women's role in health maintenance. Presented below is an analysis of the indigenous concept of health, which is based on the author's understanding of the relation of people to place. It is suggested that women see health, happiness and harmony as intimately intertwined. Their health-maintaining ceremonies, in the past, as now, seek to maintain and restore harmony, happiness, and thus health.

Women have not been the passive recipients of Western-oriented medicine, nor have they lightly accepted their new health problems. They have sought to accommodate Western health practices and to elaborate old practices where appropriate and possible. However, there is no way in which they can restore the good health, happiness and harmony they enjoyed in the past. Their independent base for action has been destroyed by the loss of land over which to forage. In the past, they drew not only on a living from the country but also the confidence that they could continue to live at one with the country of their ancestors. Today women have lost the assurance that they can effectively maintain good health.

In order to situate this discussion of women's changing role in health maintenance within the context of women's lives, we begin with a brief sketch of Kaititj history and ethnography. From there, we move on to explore the indigenous concepts of health and disease, and to present illustrative case-history material that traces through the subtle shifts of emphasis in women's ceremonies. We then turn to an examination of anthropological models, generated by male-oriented anthropologists, and conclude that a fuller understanding of health and disease must allow that both men and women have in the past — as they do now — played vital roles in the maintenance of health in Aboriginal society.

THE KAITITJ OF WARRABRI

In 1954, a new home at Warrabri was chosen for the Warlpiri and Warramunga people of the Phillip Creek Native Settlement, north of Tennant Creek, where the water supply had proved inadequate. Many Kaititj and Alyawarra people, who were living on nearby cattle-stations, drifted into Warrabri in the 1960s; some took up residence, others preferred to remain mobile between settlement and cattle-station.

In 1977, approximately 650 Aborigines and 60–70 Europeans were living at Warrabri. The Europeans lived in houses situated in the settlement core, where school, hospital, police, administrative facilities, garage, store and parks were located. This service core generated some work for Aborigines, but the majority subsisted on social security payments. Most of the Aborigines lived in makeshift camps, scattered on the periphery of the settlement service core. Warlpiri and Warramunga, who numbered approximately 350, oriented their camps to the west of the settlement core, while Kaititj and Alyawarra, approximately 300 in number, located their camps to the east. Thus the spatial relations between camps reflected the divisions in the Aboriginal population: there were those who came from and camped in the east, and those who came from and camped to the west (Bell, 1980a : 141ff.). Most importantly, however, because Warrabri is Kaititj and Alyawarra country, the Warlpiri and Warramunga are considered to be interlopers. The way in which this designation impinges upon health is discussed below.

For several generations, the Kaititj have lived in contact with, though not under the direct control of, Europeans. The Barrow Creek telegraph station, eighty kilometres south of Warrabri, established in 1872, deep in the heart of Kaititj country, provided the first sustained contact with Europeans for Aborigines living in that area. Mining activity, pastoral development and construction workers have, over the last hundred years, provided further experience of European culture for the Kaititj (Hartwig, 1965 : 259–80).

Colonization of Kaititj country has been violent. On two occasions, government parties sought out Kaititj as responsible for the loss of European lives. In 1874, a dispute over rations culminated in an Aboriginal attack on Barrow Creek telegraph station, where two whites were killed. In 1928, two whites were killed in the Coniston area. Scores if not hundreds of Aborigines, many of whom were Kaititj, lost their lives in the savage retributions that followed these incidents (Hartwig, 1960).

Pastoral expansion into Kaititj country from 1920 onwards has irrevocably affected the hunter-gatherer mode of subsistence. Kaititj lands have been appropriated by cattle-men; the sacred sites have been defiled. The main highway north from Alice Springs to Darwin runs right through the Devil's Marbles, a site of central importance to Kaititj. Despite these indignities and the violence of dispossession of land, the Kaititj have managed to sustain their religious ties to their land and to maintain many of their treasured sites.

"Country" is a critical dimension of identity for desert Aborigines, male and female, all of whom count themselves as the descendants of particular ancestors who wandered across the countryside in the *jukurrpa* (dreamtime). These ancestral beings created different physical features such as waterholes and rock formations, the flora and fauna. Part of their spiritual power still resides in these sites, tracks and in the country in general. For instance, Warrabri is "Dog-Dreaming", because in the *jukurrpa*, two dogs wandered through this country. The settlement site itself is, in the mythology, the place where the dogs sat down.

Living Aboriginal men and women hold a sacred trust to maintain the life-force of the countries to which they are affiliated, through both mother's and father's patriline. In Aboriginal English, one is known as an "owner" in the country of one's father and father's father and "manager" in the country of one's mother and mother's father. Both Aranda and Warlpiri terms that mark this distinction are in use by the Kaititj of Warrabri. In Warlpiri, one speaks of *kirda* (owner) and *kurdungurla* (manager), while in Aranda one adds a suffix to the names of the country: *aljirra* (dreaming) to the mother's country and *arinya* (belonging) to the father's country. The division of labour between owner and manager is such that members of the owning patriclan call upon the children of the senior women of their clan to act as managers in the ritual maintenance of the country. In this way, ritual knowledge and responsibility are spread through several patriclans. Ritual reciprocity between manager and owner pervades ritual organization and enactment, so that owners on one occasion will be managers on another.

Both men and women draw on their dreamtime heritage in the performance of rituals that celebrate the central values of their society, but each does so in a way appropriate to his or her sex. Some women's ceremonies, closed to men and children, ritualize women's life crises: birth, menarche. There are other more elaborate women's rituals, *yawalyu*, which celebrate ties to land and which, on occasions, men and children may attend.

Although women spend but few years of their lives in the demanding task of child-rearing, the motif of a woman as nurturer is a metaphor for women's role in many *yawalyu* ceremonies. The significance and broad themes of these rituals have been inadequately understood by male-oriented anthropologists, who have focused on men's spectacular rituals, and dismissed women's rituals as of concern to women only (see Maddock, 1972 : 155). In *yawalyu*, women are acting as nurturers of country, people and human relationships; as we shall see, this is most important in women's concept of harmonious relations and therefore well-being.

A striking feature of the life-history material collected from Kaititj women was the amount of time they had spent in their youth in contact with the country of their forebears. The effect of dislocation of people from country is thus not as marked for the Kaititj of Warrabri as for the Warlpiri, who are many miles from their own country. In my experience gained during eighteen months fieldwork in 1976–78 at Warrabri, these Kaititj women were actively engaged in ritual activity concerning the maintenance and celebration of their land and had little time to be bored. This strong basis for identity is critical to an understanding of women's perception of their role in health maintenance and the reality of women's health.

It will be argued that Kaititj women are responding to the changes wrought by contact in distinctive and deliberate ways. Unlike the Warlpiri, who also live at Warrabri, the Kaititj are not far removed from their country. Their identity is constantly renewed by their contact with their country, their pride in this continuing relationship evident in their daily lives. They can afford to reject European lifestyles, for their own still provides support and meaning.

ABORIGINAL PERSPECTIVES ON HEALTH: PEOPLE, PLACE AND PRACTICE

Aboriginal medical practice and classification of disease are sensitive to shifts in mood and situation: conflict between members of a community or transgressions of the law are considered injurious to smooth social and religious relations. Because a healthy individual or community is one in harmony with others and the world of the *jukurrpa*, Aboriginal health practitioners seek to maintain an existing state of good health or to re-establish harmony and thereby restore good health. Underpinning the indigenous concept of good health is an equilibrium model of society backed by the dogma of dreaming, which Aborigines vehemently assert exists at the level of lived reality. This conscious model of stasis masks the actual experience of people who, in their daily lives in a world of rapid change, are constantly engaged in power plays and negotiations.

Social relationships, especially those between men and women, are in a constant state of flux because, beneath the claims that men do men's business and women do women's business, is the tension generated by the unresolved power politics *between* men and women. Maintaining a semblance of unchanging continuity in the past required constant adjustment and accommodation, but in the face of the dramatic upheavals of the past century, the strain has increased.

The roles made available to Aboriginal women by the predominantly male colonial society of the Northern Territory are restrictive. Women have lost the independence they once enjoyed in their hunting and gathering activities, which made them substantially independent of the men. Women are now dependent on social security payments, which do not recognize women as independent household heads unless they are without a husband (Bell, 1980a : 165–72; Hamilton, 1975 : 173). Aboriginal women's mothering roles, and the ritual elaborations of these roles, are held in low esteem by white frontier society, which allowed Aboriginal women to become domestic labourers and sexual partners (Bell, 1980b : 241ff.). Women's critical role in decision-making also has been denied and ignored by whites who have vested authority in the predominantly male councils, which are playing an increasingly important role in the management of settlements (Bell and Ditton, 1980 : 11–12). Aboriginal men have taken advantage of this situation to advance their claims to greater control over women and the resources available on settlements. Women thus have been further marginalized.

In retrospect, Kaititj women state they were competent nurturers of people and country, and that in this role they were enhanced as women. Today Kaititj women refer to Warrabri as a "sickness place" and comment upon the good health they enjoyed in the past. Settlement sickness is juxtaposed to bush health and women often will comment that they were never sick in the bush. Indeed, one remedy for a lingering illness is time in the bush, away from the contaminating influence of the settlement. For Kaititj, there are few happy associations with the growth of Warrabri as a linguistically and culturally mixed settlement. Obviously time away from the pressures and tensions of Warrabri is beneficial, but Warrabri is considered a "sickness place" for reasons other than the stress of life in a heterogeneous community. It was, for instance, an unfortunate choice of a site for a settlement. Various ritual codes were violated, and continued to be so following the establishment of the settlement.

In selecting Warrabri as a site, government officials were guided by such criteria as the availability of water or land that pastoralists might not want. Unfortunately, they did not seek the permission of the Kaititj spokespersons of the country, who were affronted when Warlpiri people were moved to the settlement area. To further compound this error, the unfortunate Aboriginal "front guy" who was consulted, did not have the authority to sanction Warlpiri settlement in his country and died shortly after the move. Twenty years later, Kaititj Aborigines claim that he died of worry and the knowledge that he had transgressed. Warlpiri have paid heavily in cash and ritual exchange items for their residence at Warrabri, and there are still disputes generated by the tensions between the holders of the country and the interlopers.

Unfortunately, the incidents surrounding the settlement of Warrabri impinged little upon the consciousness of white officials, who continued to behave as if they were exempt from the strictures of Aboriginal law and its punishments. An oft-repeated tale, told by Kaititj with some pride, is of the policeman who attempted to rid Warrabri of its dog scourge by rounding up and removing the diseased dogs from Warrabri and then destroying them some distance away from the settlement core. This violated a sacred trust of the Kaititj and Alyawarra at Warrabri, to care for dogs and never to kill them.

Because Warrabri is dog-dreaming, all children born at Warrabri have an interest in dog-dreaming; the lives of children and dogs are inexorably linked. In the *jukurrpa*, dogs scratched and today children also scratch. It is said if dogs are destroyed children will sicken and die. After the policeman had destroyed the dogs, the old people predicted that children would become ill, and indeed they did. In order to restore harmony, the men took the policeman to the bush to reveal to him something of the power of dog-dreaming. As a consequence, dogs are no longer destroyed by whites at Warrabri. Dogs may thus continue to scratch, as do the children. Aborigines have since suggested that a veterinarian would be an appropriate answer to new health problems created by dogs.

Further tales that link behaviour, location and health, concern sorcery accusations. When the Warlpiri and Warramunga were moved from Phillip Creek to Warrabri, the old people promised the government and the mission that they would leave all their "bad magic" behind. But, say the Kaititj, one old Warlpiri man, Jangala,[2] brought it with him. The Kaititj believe that Jangala's grandfather, father and now his son all have caused trouble for people. This Warlpiri power to harm is based on their rights in and access to certain mythology associated with Rain-Dreaming. At Phillip Creek, Jangala had used his powers in order to reinforce his claims to certain women. He threatened illness if they refused him. With an ever-increasing population at Warrabri, Jangala's scope to harm women increased dramatically. No longer content merely to harry women who stood in the correct marriage relationship with him, he extended his activities to married women and women over whom he had no claim at all. In a period of one week at Warrabri, this man was believed to have caused three women to suffer.

The first, an introspective Kaititj/Anmatjirra woman, who worked in the school, was in a very distressed state for some time. Jangala had made a "pass" at her at school, but she had thought him merely to be a work friend, for he also held a position in the school. She then began to have recurrent dreams in which images of *ngapa* (water) appeared. Finally, she confided these dreams to several older Warlpiri men, who recognized the work of Jangala.

In another case, the man performed certain rituals that focused on the Warramunga mother of a girl he wished to marry (i.e. his mother-in-law). At the same time, another young Kaititj woman, whom he fancied, was suffering with a paralysed arm. Like the other woman, these two reported having *ngapa* dreams, although each dream was different. The old Warlpiri men met and decided that Jangala should remove the evil from the women. All but the first woman completely recovered. She moved to Tennant Creek in an attempt to get away from Jangala, after unsuccessfully appealing to her relatives at Ti-tree, two hundred kilometres south of Warrabri, and the local Warrabri council to assist her. Several months later, she had completely recovered.

Communities and individuals lack good health for many reasons. At the most general level, women speak of the times of "troubles" and state that if these can be ended, good health will ensue. "Troubles" may be anything from a family fight, a sudden death, an unexplained accident, a sorcery accusation or an accumulation of persistent but minor incidents of ill-fortune for a family or camp. "Troubles" do not include issues associated with the European world, such as money worries, the need for car repairs, nor a child's school performance, although people do worry about these issues.

During a time of "troubles", there is a moratorium on travel, because it is considered to be too dangerous to move about until the source of the "troubles" is located and treated. It is a time of self- and social examination, and criticism of the behaviour of one's self and others that may have occasioned the misfortune. It is a time when sorcery accusations proliferate and old arguments are revived. Thus within the domain of health, we need to include not only the *ngangkayi* (traditional healers) but also broadly based concepts of who are the patients and what constitutes modes of diagnosis and treatment. As good health has ultimately to do with good social relationships, it is essential that we examine how these are maintained. In the cases of the three women mentioned, the old men explained the problem and began its resolution. It was the relationship to certain dreamings that gave them the power and knowledge to act in this way.

SETTLEMENT HEALTH PRACTICES

Most settlement hospitals appear to be conceived of by Aborigines as female domains, as an extension of women's caring roles in the past, and in a sense this is supported by the appointment of white female nursing staff. Men may visit and receive treatment, but they generally do not work in the hospitals, nor do they gather in the shade around the hospital, as do the women, to rest and exchange news. In 1977, in the hospital at Warrabri, there were two nursing sisters employed by the Health Department and several Aboriginal health workers, who were receiving literacy and basic health care training. The degree of responsibility given to the Aboriginal health workers depends on the personality, age and maturity of the health workers and the nursing sisters. Health Department policies with regard to training and health worker education also intrude. On certain settlements in Central Australia, traditional healers and Western practice exist side by side. At Warrabri, the *ngangkayi* may be consulted by health personnel, but this practice is not institutionalized (Elkin, 1977 : 158–59). If people wish to visit the *ngangkayi* at Warrabri, they usually do so in the camp.

Certain literacy skills are required if Aboriginal health workers are to assume real responsibility in health care programmes. Frequently, young girls chosen as health workers because they have the literacy skills, do not have the status in their own community to exercise the authority required of the really autonomous health workers. Also young white women assume positions of authority as nursing sisters on settlements, which is hard for older people, especially older men, to accept. Through the health worker education programmes organized by the Health Department, older women are being given the necessary training to cope with the demands of the position. Health worker schemes also are attempting to integrate aspects of both medical systems by demystifying Western medicine, while at the same time encouraging incorporation of Aboriginal practices. A new and growing respect for Aboriginal values also is apparent among some medical personnel as they have come to realize the depth of knowledge and concern that Aborigines demonstrate in times of illness.

However, the autonomy that women once enjoyed in the domain of health has not been regained through participation in health worker schemes. These proceed cautiously; authority and responsibility are delegated slowly. Certain critical skills are withheld, as the Warrabri people found to their chagrin in late 1977. On this occasion, the Health Department of Alice Springs decided to withdraw all nursing sisters and certain medicines from Warrabri because there had been a series of attacks and two alleged attempted rapes of white women by Aboriginal men. The Health Department feared for the safety of their nurses. Although many old and bitter arguments were aired in public, in the open confrontation between the health personnel and the Aboriginal people at Warrabri, one taunt from the women recurred. "We have been trained, but we can't take over," the women challenged the officials. "We can't give injections. Our old people will die if they can't have the medicine they now need." "Why are we being punished?" asked one younger woman. "What have we done? We do not rape white men. We need the medicines." The men were more concerned to assume responsibility for the wayward youths and assure the white officials that there would be no more attacks. The women were more interested in the area for which they assumed responsibility. That they had, since contact with white Australians, been reduced to a state of dependency and were being kept there, was clear to most women that day.

HEALTH CEREMONIES

Crises of Life Ceremonies

Catherine Berndt (Berndt and Berndt, 1946 : 15), writing of the cattle-stations in the north-west of the Northern Territory in 1944–46, noted that following contact with Europeans, women's ceremonies are the first to disintegrate. At Warrabri, it also is true that the major crises of life ceremonies for women have been almost entirely usurped by white institutions. Childbirth now occurs in hospital and first menstruation is most likely when a girl is at school. Other traditionally female responsibilities also have been undermined on settlements. For example, the health of babies is now monitored by health authorities. It is suggested that not only has this created a situation in which women no longer control their own fertile lives but it also has engendered a feeling of inadequacy in women. The loss of control and the damage to a woman's self-respect have scarcely been noted by anthropologists, who have considered women's activities to be small-scale and of little consequence. Women's ceremonies have been relegated to the realm of the magical, the secular and the domestic hearth.

Because birth and early child care are exclusively female affairs, where strict rules and practices are observed, women in the past were able to exercise control over their own bodies and fertile lives (Cowlishaw, 1977). If a child was born to a young mother, too close to a sibling, or obviously deformed, it was the decision of the mother to practise infanticide. This is not to imply that women did not love and cherish their children; it is merely an example of their right to decide which child would live at birth. Although actual birth now nearly always occurs in hospital, as soon as the mother leaves, the women take her and the child away into the bush, where they perform certain rituals to ensure the health and growth of the child and the renewed strength of the mother. The use of herbal preparations and plants in the childbirth rituals is the only consistent use of plants (for health and curing) I observed at Warrabri. Women have extensive knowledge of plants and usage, but they tend to discuss rather than use the plants. "Aspirin and Vicks are more powerful," they say, "but we like to visit the country and collect the plants too."

As neither childbirth nor first menstruation can be timed to occur in a season of plenty, as can initiation, these ceremonies have to concern those female relatives who might be present in the family camps. It is interesting to note that women state that now, as in the past, it was their "mother's mother" who attended them in birth. For this to be so, the couple must have lived with, or close by to the wife's grandmother.

In the past, formal rituals to limit the size of families were in the hands of men. However, the practice of extensive breast-feeding, the segregation of the sexes, the later sexual maturity of girls in the past, the tolerance of a high infant mortality rate and infanticide, all supported the male ritual statements that large families were undesirable, but left the actual physical controls in the hands of women. The shift to a sedentary lifestyle has altered many of these patterns and women are now bearing many children, at a younger age and closer together. Sickly children are surviving, but spend many months in hospital, away from their families. They return to their communities as outsiders and with younger siblings who require attention. Younger women are beginning to seek contraceptive advice, but are still somewhat bewildered by their increased fertility and fecundity.

Older women comment that the law is no longer being upheld.

In the past, children could not have been born to mothers so young, they insist. Mindful of the experience of other fieldworkers (see Goodale, 1971 : 136), and fearful of a withering reply, nevertheless this subject was pursued with one close friend, who was asked why such young girls were having babies today. The answer was, that in the past, girls did not marry until "their breasts hung down". To the question: "But what about the young unmarried girls who play around?", indicating one young mother whom the women had been discussing, came the reply: "In the past, girls slept in one place and the boys in another. There was no 'humbug' then."

At first menstruation, women celebrated the attainment of sexual maturity of a female child, who now could assume new responsibilities. Although these were relatively small-scale rituals, they were acknowledged as areas of female autonomy and authority, with special importance for members of the girl's matriline. For the mother of the girl, it marked the beginning of a new stage in her role as a mother-in-law, and for her mother, a realization of arrangements made for her daughter some fifteen years previously (Bell, 1980a : 335–51).

Yawalyu

During the past fifty years, women's health activities have undergone a subtle shift, from those organized within the matriline and focused on the individual to wider land-based (*yawalyu*) rituals, based on the *kirda-kurdungurlu* relationship. This reflects the interaction of women's perceptions of their necessarily changing role as nurturers and the changing milieu in which they live. The focus has shifted from the relationship of the individual with the spiritual world to the relationships between groups and their spiritual world. Given the broad-based concept of health, this new emphasis is an accurate assessment of the troubles that are at present causing ill-health. Problems now occur within the large heterogeneous settlement community, not within the smaller homogeneous family group.

Yawalyu ceremonies are not solely concerned with health, although this is one of the main themes and stated purposes of women in staging one. *Yawalyu* evoke the three major themes of land, love and health. The imagery of these interlocking themes is embedded in the central symbols of fat, colour and the attendant emotional, physical and psychological states. Two of the most important dreamings of the Kaititj women at Warrabri are *ngapa* (rain) and *yawaki* (bush-berry), which focus upon three major sites: *Waaka*, *Wakulpu* and *Karlukarlu*. Although many other dreaming tracks criss-cross and link these sites, it is in the travels of the ancestral women of the Rain and Bush-berry Dreamings and in the final going-down into the ground of the essence of the *yawaki* (bush-berry) ancestor, that the themes of health find clearest expression.

From the red of *Karlukarlu* (Devil's Marbles) rises the power of life-force and blood. Through massage with fat, prepared during a performance of a *yawalyu* for the country around Devil's Marbles, the power can be activated by women. To this redness is juxtaposed the whiteness of rain and lightning as it flashes dangerously overhead. This whiteness is disturbed and challenged by the brilliance of the colours of the rainbow men, who pursue women in the area. With Bush-berry is associated all that is black in the natural world. In his journey from Waaka to Wakulpu, Bush-berry is accompanied by his faithful companions, the little birds called *Yirlpadirlpadirlpa*. Mourning, the devotion of his bird friends, and correct ritual relations between manager and owner are portrayed in the travels of Bush-berry. In both dreamings, fat is the medium through which the power of the dreaming is transformed and transmitted by the women who own and manage the ceremonies and country.

Fat is the central symbol of women's ritual, in that it links the major themes of love, health and land. While the dreamtime heroes pioneered the country, they rubbed themselves with fat and admired the beauty and redness of their bodies. To glow with health is to be as one who is covered with fat. A lover cannot help but be attracted by the glowing good health of the body that reflects contentment and the strength of one who had access to country of one's dreaming. As bullock fat is now readily available, it is possible to grease and paint more bodies more often than in the past, when one relied on emu, goanna or witchetty fat. Fat is seen as imparting strength and requires special ritual attention in all women's health-maintaining and curing rituals.

During these rituals, which may vary from a short singing of the country and preparation of ritual paraphernalia, to a three-day marathon of dancing, singing, teaching and displays, women remove themselves from the main camp area and usually use the women's ritual area. As with the men, there is a division of labour based on the owner/manager relationship discussed above, but the women who are present also may emphasize other aspects of their relationships to each other.

In analysing data, those songs have been isolated that have to do specifically with health as if they constituted a discrete corpus of health chants. These songs occur within the context of *yawalyu* performances of country in general. There is, however, some support for this classification in the minds and practice of the Warrabri

Kaititj. Health songs that have to do with a particular condition such as a swelling, sore, pain or temperature are said to be "properly old ones" or "properly dear ones". They are thus distinguished from other songs sung during a *yawalyu* performance that may have health as its focus, but also concern country in a general sense. When the women sing these specific songs for health, they bathe with water for swellings and fevers, and massage with fat for pain and weakness. At a higher level of generality, curing songs are specified by a gesture that involves a pushing-away action. In this action, the women hold their cupped hands before themselves and shuffle the hands outwards from their bodies, thus signifying the sending out and bestowing of power. They also use this gesture when singing specific health chants and certain land songs that have to do with the restoration of well-being. It is a gesture that is said to be for those who are *murrumurru* (sick). Women therefore clearly distinguish in several ways songs that have to do with health and curing.

As areas in which women could express their powers and control over their bodies (birth, menarche) have declined and been undermined by Western institutions, other modes of expressing concern, care and communication have been elaborated and emphasized. This involves, as stated, a delicate interplay of women's perceptions of what is their role (to care, nurture and restore harmony) and the pragmatics of the situation (hospitals, group structure, settlement location). Women have recognized that their ill-health has more to do with conditions of the settlement than with their individual behaviours and that powerful remedies therefore must be sought to restore the balance. They have responded by incorporating certain elements of the individual healing rituals within the larger group-based ceremonies.

Increasingly, women are drawing upon *yawalyu* rituals, but all the various ritual forms to which women have been turning in their pursuit of good health, can be seen as falling along a continuum. At one end are the individual-oriented ceremonies, organized within the matriline and primarily concerned with crises of life, and at the other are the group-oriented ceremonies that involve women as owners and managers. Focus, scope, structure and content all reflect women's changing role and status.

CHANGING CEREMONIES

In the following three cases, the changes and continuities in women's role in health maintenance are demonstrated. In the first two cases, women who are *kirda* and *kurdungurlu* prepare the fat while singing the country of Rain-Dreaming. This fat is then taken to the camp of the patient, where massage (and perhaps more singing) occurs. In the second case, the specific songs are sung for fat and ochre, which are prepared in the presence of the patient. These activities are concentrated within the matriline, but other relationships are involved. The structural principle underlying the dreamings being used in the health ritual is that of *kirda* to *kurdungurlu*.

In the third case, the women sang for the individual, but the songs then were incorporated into a wider celebration of country. Once the song for the particular condition had been sung, the women then continued with the cycle until they had reached a point where they were satisfied the patient had absorbed the power. On these occasions there may be more than one patient and small children often are brought forward to be painted. In the most complex form, as described later for case four, the women staged a full *yawalyu*, with dancing, ritual paraphernalia and exchange of gifts or knowledge. Although it must remain supposition, I believe this elaborate form and mode of expressing concern with ill-health and attempting to restore good health is now sought more often than it was in the past. As women find their powers undermined, they are turning to the more powerful, spectacular rituals, in the hope that, by correctly observing the law, their health will improve.

Case One: Jakamarra

> Old Jakamarra had been ill for some time, but had only recently been brought to Warrabri by his concerned relatives from Barrow Creek. They hoped that the Nungarrayi of Warrabri (his nieces, close "sisters' daughters") could help restore this man to good health. In their own ritual area, the women prepared fat and red ochre, which was formed into a ball and taken to the camp of Jakamarra by Nakamarra and Nungarrayi women (i.e. "sisters" and "sisters' daughters"). After a brief discussion with Jakamarra's wife, the women massaged the patient in much the same way as does the *ngangkayi*, but the culmination of the massage was the painting of the feet, through the soles of which the illness could later escape. Although the visit lasted only about fifteen minutes, Jakamarra knew that the women were working for him before they arrived, and that they would continue to do so after the visit, until he improved. Later that evening, he drank tea for the first time for weeks, and the next day began eating.

It is not unusual for people to seek health care from professionals who do not belong to their own community. In the case above, the man was closely related, but women have asked to be taken to places as far away as Areyonga, south of Alice Springs, in order to seek particularly powerful *ngangkayi* or a more appropriate dreaming for a particular condition than the dreamings they may use. In the case of Jakamarra, he was cured, the women said, because he heard the songs of his country sung. It was a restoration, a "putting-in-touch with" process, whereby he experienced, through the women, the attachment of the dreamtime heroes as they travelled through the country and the well-being the ancestors felt in their country. The "daughters" were *kurdungurlu* for the country — that is, those who assist in the staging of rituals. They therefore were playing a dual role: firstly, as "daughters" and members of his caring matriline, and secondly, as ritual managers for his dreaming.

Case Two: Jakamarra

Another case, similar but more elaborate, and remembered as successful, is that of another Jakamarra. This incident took place thirty years ago. Today, the man lives at Warrabri. He is an unusually tall and muscular man, but there was a time when he was so weak that he could no longer stand.

> At the time of Jakamarra's ill-health, the people were living at Wauchope, fifty kilometres north of Warrabri, on the wolfram mines. All the Napanangka (his "mothers") gathered to assist in his treatment. Together, in the bush away from the camp of the man, the five "mothers" prepared a mixture of goanna and witchetty fat. The ritual involved singing over various pieces of hair string, which, once prepared, were taken to the man's camp. He was stripped and dressed with hair string.
>
> In retelling the story, the women emphasize that the men were powerless to do anything. "They just sat there worrying." The women were in charge and directed the men as to which articles of clothing were to be removed and which not. Before they began, even Jakamarra was convinced he would die. The women massaged his head, shoulders, hands and feet, with special attention to the navel, for which there are powerful health and love designs. At this stage, the women were using fat only.
>
> They kept vigil all night as they sang the dreaming that infuses the country with strength and colour. In the morning, they again massaged Jakamarra, but this time with a mixture of red ochre and fat. A white head-band was substituted for the hair string around his head. This was a symbol of purity as well as attractiveness. All day he lay in the men's camp. In the afternoon, he began to feel better and announced that the next day he would go hunting, which he did. Everyone was happy to see him better and moving around. According to the women, he is now protected from that illness for the rest of his life.

When the women were asked about the possibility of a *ngangkayi* treating the man, the answer was that no *ngangkayi* was present at Wauchope years ago, and that in any case, his condition required the treatment given by the women, by his "mothers".

In the next case, the use of the *yawalyu* to cure the woman was structured differently from the two previous examples. A particular song was required, and it had to be sung in the context of the country to which it belonged. The women worked from the particular (i.e. the condition of the patient) to the general (i.e. association with country) in attempting to restore health. This performance required the presence of the *kirda* and *kurdungurlu*, which was facilitated by the concentration of people at Warrabri. The Jakamarra at Wauchope could not have expected to be treated by this scale of ritual, because there were too few people living in the mines to be able to stage such a *yawalyu*.

Case Three: Napurrula

Napurrula recently had undergone gynaecological surgery, but was still retaining fluid and was in some discomfort. She herself was a *ngangkayi*, but it was the women of the Nampijinpa-Nangala semi-moiety who, in consultation with a Nungarrayi, the *kurdungurlu* for those dreamings, assisted her. All this took place in the presence of her Napurrula sister. Women may ask each other for *yawalyu*, or for arm blood (a potent medicine), and no doubt other items to do with health, but it is generally a joint decision of the patient and the *kirda* and *kurdungurlu* to stage a *yawalyu*.

> The group assembled and sang the specific songs to ease the pain and reduce the swellings. This involved two dreamings: rain, to reduce the swelling, and bush-berry, to impart strength. The women sang of the ancestral women who rubbed fat into hair string to make them feel strong again. They then invoked, with singing, the presence of the *ngangkayi* familiar, so he could enter the woman and remove the source of the pain. Once that was achieved, the women moved to rain dreaming, to sing the wound shut. All the while, they were massaging and painting Napurrula with a design that is particularly powerful in restoring good health and good spirits. Aspects of the ceremony are even considered a little provocative by the women, in that the designs and songs have sexual overtones.
>
> During this ceremony, two other ailing women with long-standing conditions were painted and massaged. Children were also painted, but the major focus of the ceremony was on the pain and swelling of Napurrula.

This ceremony incorporated the emphasis on the individual being cared for by members of her own matriline, with the structural

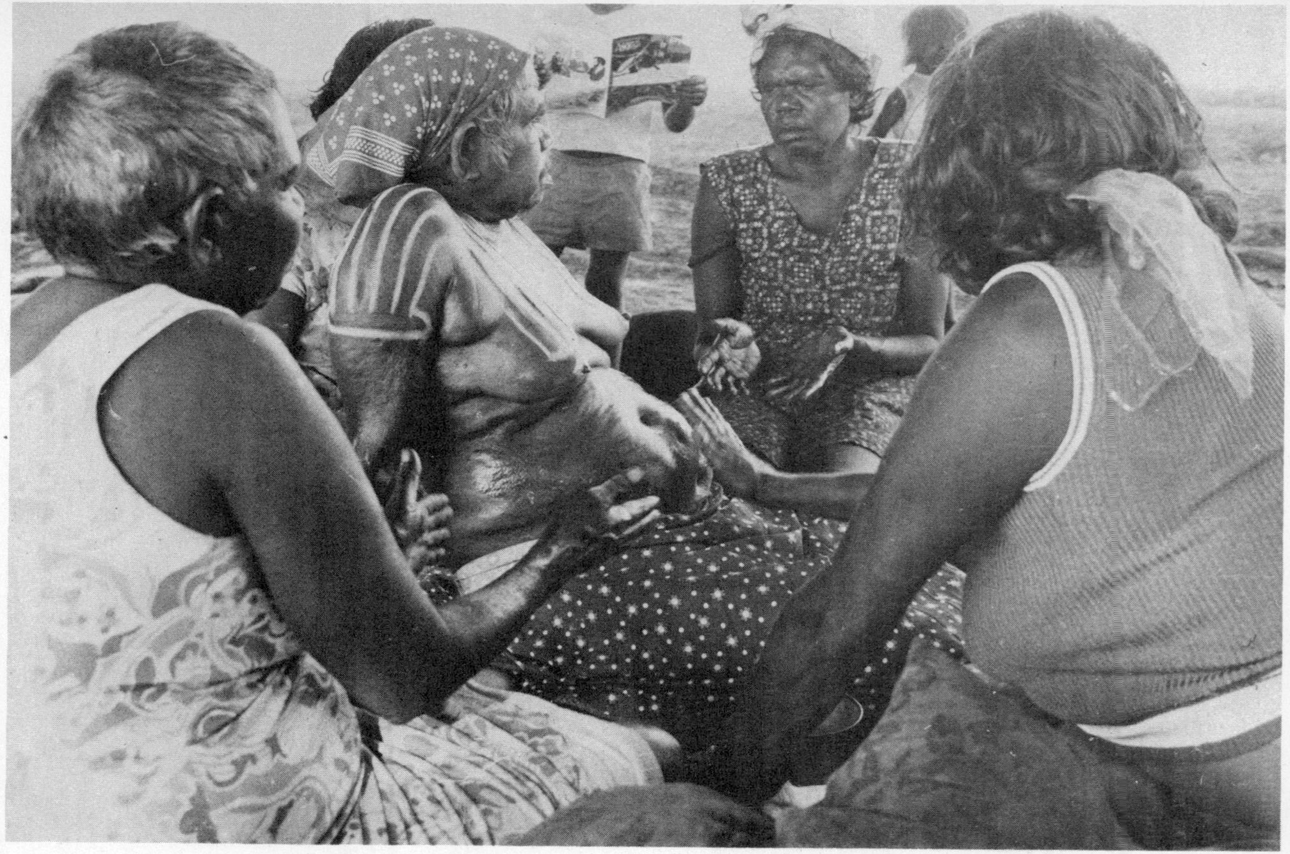

Napurrula is painted and massaged, to ease the pain and reduce the swelling.

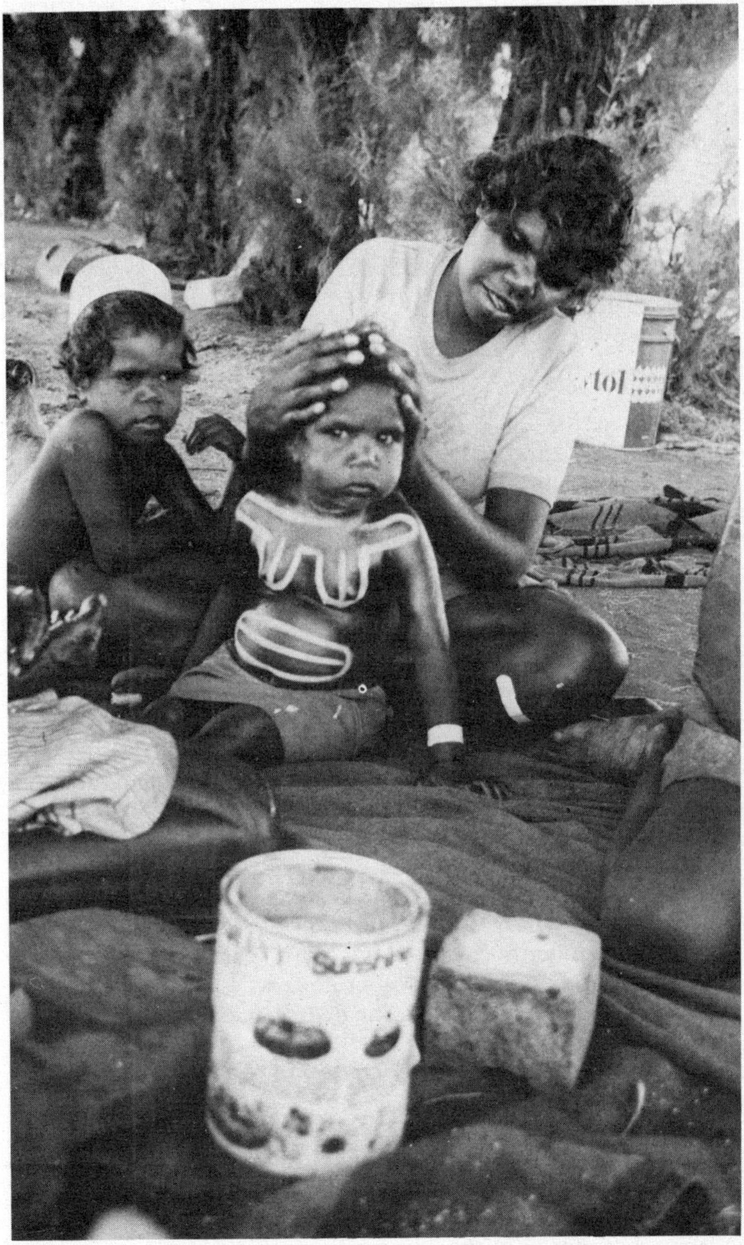

A child was also painted during the ceremony.

relationship of *kirda* to *kurdungurlu*. The children who were painted belonged to those women present at the ceremony. In some cases, this meant that the children were *kirda* or *kurdungurlu*, but in others, they were neither. Once again in this ceremony we can see an incorporation of smaller family rituals, focused on the caring matriline, into the structure of the larger land-based ceremonies based on the *kirda–kurdungurlu* relationship.

In the fourth case described below, the shift from the family and matriline to the ritual group is complete. Although in this case "sisters" help "mothers", they refer to each other as *kirda* and *kurdungurla*, not in the kin terms of mother and daughter, or sister to sister.

Case Four: Nungarrayi

Nungarrayi is the daughter of an extremely important Japaljarri, *kirda* for Kangaroo-Dreaming. He had taught his daughter the stories of other dreamings for which he was also part-*kirda*. This woman is held in high esteem in Willowra, Tennant Creek and at Warrabri, for she is considered to be extremely knowledgeable and powerful. Through her father, she is *kirda* for Snake-Dreaming near Willowra. She also holds the songs and stories for a Honey-Dreaming site, *Lilpunju*, and through her conception site, Spear-Dreaming at *Kurlarda Kurlangu*. She is the chief *kurdungurlu* for the Nampijinpa–Nangala dreamings of rain and bush-berry. She has two older sons, who have been through initiation ceremonies, and a younger daughter by her second husband.

Her love rituals, which secured her present husband, are considered powerful and envied by many other women at Warrabri, who alternatively blame this woman for troubles in their love lives or ask her to work for them. Her own marriage has been a stormy love-hate relationship, with passionate and jealous fights. Her mother-in-law, Napangardi, is closer in age to Nungarrayi than Nungarrayi is to her husband, who is many years her junior. Added to this, the mother-in-law is a querulous woman, who constantly interferes in her son's marriage. She had been asked to leave several camps because of her temper, and finally the daughter-in-law and husband moved to the other side of Warrabri, to avoid her meddling ways.

Nungarrayi is very aware of the power and potential danger of the love rituals she owns, and frequently cautions other women not to sing songs that are not correctly theirs. She herself is very careful to observe all precautions to control the powers, but her mother-in-law accuses her of starting all the fights that take place. The husband does little to check his mother and, after returning from one spree in town, accused his wife of adultery, and in spite of her pleading, beat her unmercifully. She left him and refused to return until he promised to stop drinking. This he did, but women outside her group say that she is sick all the time because of his ill-treatment.

Nungarrayi had been generally ill for some time and had sought assistance from the hospital, the ***ngangkayi*** and the women of her own dreaming group. Finally, the old ***ngangkayi***, a classificatory son (i.e. within the matriline) was called in and prescribed ***yawalyu***.

It was a close daughter and a "mother's father's sister" of Nungarrayi who told of the beginning of her "troubles". Several years back, when the mother, son and wife had been at Willowra for initiation business, Nungarrayi had fought with her mother-in-law and drawn blood. Napangardi took the blood in a handkerchief to several Nampijinpa "sisters-in-law" at Willowra. (The sick Nungarrayi is ***kurdungurlu*** for the dreamings of these Willowra women.) The rituals that the Willowra women did with the blood are said to have caused Nungarrayi's illness. The only way for her to recover was to appease the Willowra women with a gift in exchange for the blood.

The organization that preceded the Willowra trip took over a month, and it became evident that the Nungarrayi women were going to use this occasion to settle many old scores. Women have restricted access to cars, so they cannot visit as readily as men. The women maximized the opportunity to restore as many harmonious relationships as possible. The trip to Willowra became a complex of relationships, beliefs about health, personal knowledge, dreamings and demography.

Although the two days of dancing, singing, painting, teaching and exchanges centred on the Rain- and Bush-berry Dreaming of the Kaititj women of Warrabri, the revelation and gift of the knowledge of Snake- and Honey-Dreaming to the Willowra women also was effected. Nungarrayi was at the centre of proceedings, but all the Nampijinpa and Nungarrayi women of Willowra participated.

The activities that were strictly health-related were short and spectacular. Nungarrayi, after she had presented the dreamings of snake and honey to the Willowra women, also gave them the sacred paraphernalia of Bush-berry to look after for some years. They then painted, massaged and exorcised the spirits from her. The separation of fat and colour, as in the Jakamarra cases, was also followed by the Willowra women, but Nungarrayi assured them if their work was not good, she would "hot it up a bit" with Rainbow-Dreaming. Once all the gift exchanges and dancing were finished, the Willowra women painted Nungarrayi with a Willowra-owned design and thus completed the singing of country.

Throughout the rituals held at Willowra, the organization both reflected and was spoken of in terms of ***kirda*** and ***kurdungurlu.*** In presenting Snake-Dreaming, Nungarrayi was ***kirda*** to the Willowra women, who were receiving it as her joint ***kirda.*** In fact, they also were full or close sisters, but that was not the aspect of the relationship that was stressed. It was not the kin relationship that was important in these rituals but the power of ownership of women who also were sisters. In presenting the bush-berry sacra, Nungarrayi was ***kurdungurlu*** to the Willowra ***kirda.*** These women were related as "mother" and "daughter", but again that was not the aspect of the relationship that was stressed. In giving away so much ritual property, Nungarrayi hoped that the jealous fights would cease and that her health would improve once harmony was restored.

In presenting these case-studies, it is argued that, despite the changes of the past one hundred years, Aboriginal women have continued to assert that they are nurturers of country, people, and social relationships. Within this analysis, it is impossible to dismiss women's activities in the domain of health maintenance as merely "growing up" children and applying a few herbal remedies. Women, in order to maintain good health, are staging ceremonies that focus on health at the cosmic level of restoration of harmony and happiness. This is so because women have the rights in the country from which they derive power and for which they hold a sacred trust. It is this aspect of their heritage that they are increasingly emphasizing.

CEREMONIAL INTERDEPENDENCE: MALE AND FEMALE, OLD AND NEW

Women's role in health maintenance has been overlooked and trivialized, because women have not been recognized as owners of country, as ritually important to the whole society, and further, the domain of health has been too narrowly defined. The focus has been on the role of the healer rather than on the way in which health is maintained over a period of time. Before turning to an examination of why this should be so, one final case-study will be presented, in which the interdependence and complementarity of male and female roles and the accommodation of Western medical practice in maintaining health are apparent.

Case Five: Nampijinpa

Nampijinpa was an astute young person, who enjoyed caring for other people's children, but was, she said, terrified of having children herself. She was married to a man who already had a large family by his first wife. Her "mothers" and "sisters" had been concerned about her for some time, because she was not eating, was listless and breathing rapidly. The women massaged and painted her, but this was not producing the hoped-for results. The hospital had not been able to relieve the symptoms either. Although at Warrabri she had the support of close "mothers" and "sisters", she wanted her actual mother, who lived at Willowra, nearly three hundred kilometres away. Nampijinpa summoned the mother by telegram. (It is not unusual for people to travel many hundreds of kilometres to visit sick relatives or to seek attention.)

> At dusk one day, at the request of Nampijinpa, the women of her mother's camp held a conference. The patient was examined and it was decided that rituals of a dreaming other than those held by the Kaititj at Warrabri were needed. The "mothers" had tried with their own *ngapa* dreaming rituals, but they now prescribed the diamond dove-dreaming of a Warlpiri Napurrula woman. It was hoped that this dreaming might be successful in restoring the woman to good health. (To visit this Napurrula meant crossing the east–west line that divides Warrabri into those who come from the west and those who come from the east. Such a crossing of boundaries is not unusual in cases of illness.)
>
> Napurrula, in consultation with the "mothers" and "sisters" of the patient, decided the services of the *ngangkayi* were necessary. Nampijinpa then visited the healer, who examined and massaged her in much the same way as her own "mothers" and "sisters" had. He could find no foreign objects to remove from her body and did not draw blood. "She needs rest and her husband," he diagnosed. The women returned to their camp, made a separate bed for the young woman and her husband and allowed the couple some privacy for the evening. Nampijinpa recovered slowly but appreciably during the following week, and later sought contraceptive advice from the hospital.

In this case, the knowledge of the *ngangkayi* far exceeded that of the normal general practitioner, and certainly that available to the settlement hospital. The diagnosis and treatment involved both Western medical practice and the knowledge and care of the members of the woman's own camp, women of another ritual group and a male *ngangkayi*. The health of Nampijinpa was the concern of her society.

Anthropological Models

Male *ngangkayi* practice possibly could be analytically opposed to female curing and peace-making procedures, in order to achieve some neat symbolic oppositions, but the foregoing discussion shows that the oppositions cannot be so starkly drawn. For in Central Australia, while the *ngangkayi* is predominantly a male role, women also may be *ngangkayi*. Also, elements of *ngangkayi* practice are incorporated in women's health maintenance activities. During ritual performance, women may summon the *ngangkayi* power, which manifests itself as a clicking in the head (Cawte, 1974 : 15; Elkin, 1977 : 23). Women also may carry the *ngangkayi* stones and, through the performance of their crises of life and *yawalyu* ceremonies, effect similar ends to that of *ngangkayi*. Men, on the other hand, stage resolution of conflict ceremonies, which restore harmony and diffuse tensions within a community (Peterson, 1970) and, as Elkin (1977), Reid (1978) and Berndt (1964) demonstrate, curing and the restoration of harmonious social relations also are part of male *ngangkayi* practice. Both men and women, in seeking to maintain health, are drawing on a shared set of values and practices.

How then are we to characterize the roles of men and women in health maintenance? On the basis of the following brief discussion of the literature on health in Aboriginal society, it is suggested that the restrictive nature of the research and the anthropological models in Aboriginal Australia have obscured the role of women in health maintenance, and in the process also have obscured the interdependence and complementarity between male and female practices in the domain of health. Rather than excluding women from the practice of medicine, it is suggested that we need to examine their contribution in terms of the indigenous concepts of good health and women's role as nurturer. All women's group ritual curing activities have to do with giving, with the infusing of the body with strength. Women attempt to restore a person to health by the gift of blood, fat or bodily secretions from underarm or eyes. In giving, women are once again acting out their nurturance role, where love, care and power are freely given. *Ngangkayi* practice, on the other hand, is essentially an individual activity, concerned more with the removal of foreign objects and alien forces from a person.

Elkin (1977 : 66), writing primarily of the 1940s (with inclusion of some more recent material in a second edition), characterized the medicine-men as those who are respected, often of outstanding personality and of "immense social significance, the psychological health of the group largely depending on their powers". In Elkin's (1977 : 12) analysis, medicine-men have skills, as well as special powers women rarely attain or possess. Women care for the minor ailments and accidents, but men have the access to the supernatural forces in the execution of their activities.

Cawte (1974 : xvii), in his comparison of coastal and desert people, argues that medicine-men's activities are directed at law and order rather than the relieving of suffering. His data on Central Australian women, who in his analysis (1974 : 144–45) cannot be doctors since they lack access to dreamtime powers, was elicited from Mrs Fleming, the wife of the missionary at Yuendumu and some of her Aboriginal women friends.

The common factor in the studies of Berndt (1964), Cawte (1974) and Elkin (1977) is that Aboriginal men are depicted as controlling the domain of health. Women may have their own business, but they do not appear as doctors and healers.

At Warrabri, it was found that women may well assume the role of *ngangkayi*. Important criteria for selection of *ngangkayi* in Central Australia, and perhaps the most critical, appear to be place in family and the dreamings upon which one may call. Should the first-born be a girl, whose younger sibling is a girl or a much younger boy, she will not only enjoy the unique position of the first-born but also the investment of dreaming knowledge from her father, not shared by subsequent siblings. Further, if she belongs to a dreaming that has important *ngangkayi* powers, she may well develop the skills and exercise the powers of *ngangkayi*. One of the constraints on women who may have received or activated the latent *ngangkayi* power is their involvement in the time-consuming and emotionally demanding task of child-rearing. As with the male practice of *ngangkayi*, it is generally older individuals who practise. These women are released from mothering duties, but they also are the women who a male ethnographer is most unlikely to contact, because most of their day is spent in the single women's camp, which is forbidden to men. Neither Cawte (1974) nor Meggitt (1955) worked closely with women on health-related issues.[3]

Elkin (1977 : 115, 124) does make passing reference to two incidents involving women doctors among the Anula and some East Kimberleys peoples. Spencer and Gillen (1899 : 465, 526) also mention women doctors and the role of women in health maintenance. However, passing reference is merely made to their training and getting of wisdom, in a fashion similar to that of their male counterparts. Their activities are not closely documented or analysed.

In Strehlow (1971 : 650–53), there are clues concerning the nature of the relationship between the sexes in Aranda health practice. Both men and women, he notes, have songs exclusive to their sex. Only women may sing the songs for women, although a brother may sit nearby, to increase the efficacy of the "charm". In form, metre and language, the songs of men and women are identical, Strehlow (1971 : 653) claims. The difference lies in the women's use of red ochre and fat, and the men's use of blood and fat. Only men may sing sacred place-names, which are taboo to women, but as

Strehlow (1971 : 653) admits, he learnt the women's songs from a man, and possibly women have other songs of which he is unaware. Certainly in the author's experience, women's secret songs are sung by the women in their own ritual area before any "treatment" occurs in a more open area.

In focusing on the activities of women that maintain health over a period of time, it is argued that underlying the changes is an enduring model of women's role, through which Aboriginal women at Warrabri achieve continuity in their rituals. It is suggested we look beyond the assertion that "nothing changes and that is how health is maintained", to examine how health is maintained through time. Rather than focus on the success and failure of a dyadic relationship, which is cast as adaptive or maladaptive (Cawte, 1974), we need to examine change, continuity and complementarity.

CONCLUSION

The role of women in the domain of health in Aboriginal society has been rendered almost invisible by the focus upon the healer and not the healed, the disease and not the context of the ill-health, the magico-religious practices and not the social-structural relationships of health to other aspects of the culture. However, it is suggested that women are acutely aware of the decline in physical health and the breakdown in social relationships. Fighting and drunkenness now disrupt their lives in a fashion unknown several generations ago. Women are aware that in the shift from a hunter-gatherer mode of subsistence to settlement life, they have suffered. Daily they are presented with tensions and sorcery accusations on a scale that could not have been sustained in the past. They have sought to repair and restore damaged bonds through their most powerful and spectacular rituals.

This resurgence of women's ritual activity has not been accompanied by a concomitant increase in the status of women. As has been argued, their autonomy has been fundamentally eroded and their relationship to land dislocated. Women's contribution to the maintenance of health in the past was within the small family group and focused upon life crisis ceremonies. It was in these rituals that women stated their importance as the makers of adult women and their control over their own bodies. Here, then, is the psychological basis for their nurturance roles: women do give birth, they do menstruate. This power and the nurturance roles associated with birth and growth are symbolized in *yawalyu* rituals.

The increased attention now being paid by women to the *yawalyu* ceremonies is both a reflection of women's perceptions of their changed circumstances and evidence of women's continuing intention to find a role in the maintenance of health and harmony. The nurturance role is now more symbolically expressed than prior to settlement life, when woman's control over the lives of the family group and bodily care and functions was more immediate and direct. Nurturance is now being stated in terms of country and relationships.

This change in emphasis does not negate the self-image of women. It does, however, partly explain women's low status on settlements, for the task they have set themselves and the means with which they seek to obtain harmony, are constrained by the male-oriented and dominated European controls and policies that govern Aboriginal affairs. The women's ceremonies that are concerned with health also are concerned with other aspects of women's role and status in Aboriginal society. Women's ceremonies often have been characterized by anthropologists as hearth-bound and their cures as domestic. Women certainly do have extensive knowledge of herbal remedies, but their activities are not restricted to the hearth. The designation by observers of "domestic" as of less importance than the male "political" roles is only possible today, when the relationships between men and women have been fundamentally altered. In the shift from a kin-based group to the emerging stratified society on settlements, women have moved from being members of an autonomous sex to being dependent and controlled. But *yawalyu* persists, albeit in a changing form and with new functions for maintaining the bonds between people and country.

NOTES

[1] Elkin (1977) writes of medicine-men, Berndt (1964) of native doctors, Reid (1978) of Aboriginal healers. I have used traditional healer, or the Warrabri Warlpiri term *ngangkayi*.

[2] Throughout the case-study material, I have used subsection (or skin) names. See Meggitt (1962 : 165–87) for a discussion of this system of social classification.

[3] Meggitt (1955 : 377) mentions in his discussion of *djanba* and medicine-men that his female informants were two young women, aged twenty and twenty-five, whereas his male informants were old men who were obviously schooled in the law.

ACKNOWLEDGEMENTS

I gratefully acknowledge the support of the Australian National University and the Australian Institute of Aboriginal Studies, which made possible my fieldwork in Central Australia. I am indebted to Janice Reid for her critical comments on the various drafts of this paper, to Doug Jervis for the photographs and to Margaret Lanigan for the typing. Finally, I wish to thank the women of Warrabri, who cared for my children and me in the field.

REFERENCES

Bell, D., 1980a. "Daughters of the Dreaming" (Ph.D. thesis, Australian National University, Canberra).

——, 1980b. "Desert Politics: Choices in the 'Marriage Market' ", in *Women and Colonization: Anthropological Perspectives*, ed. M. Etienne and E. Leacock (New York : Praeger), pp. 239–69.

——, and Ditton, P., 1980. *Law: The Old and The New: Aboriginal Women in Central Australia Speak Out* (Canberra : Aboriginal History. Distrib. by Australian National University Press).

Berndt, C. H., 1964. "The Role of Native Doctors in Aboriginal Australia", in *Magic, Faith and Healing*, ed. A. Kiev (New York : The Free Press of Glencoe), pp. 264–82.

Berndt, R. M., and Berndt, C. H., 1946. "Some Aspects of Native Labour on Northern Cattle Stations", *Aborigines Protector* 2, no. 2 : 9–18.

Cawte, J. E., 1974. *Medicine is the Law* (Honolulu : University Press of Hawaii).

Cowlishaw, G. K., 1977. "Infanticide in Aboriginal Australia", *Oceania* 48, no. 4 : 262–83.

Elkin, A. P., 1977. *Aboriginal Men of High Degree.* (St Lucia : University of Queensland Press, 2nd edn); first published 1945.

Goodale, J. C., 1971. *Tiwi Wives* (Seattle : University of Washington Press).

Hamilton, A., 1975. "Aboriginal Women: The Means of Production", in *The Other Half*, ed. J. Mercer (Ringwood : Penguin), pp. 169–79.

Hartwig, M. C., 1960. "The Coniston Killings" (B.A. (Hons) thesis, University of Adelaide).

——, 1965. "The Progress of White Settlement in the Alice Springs District and its Effect upon Aboriginal Inhabitants, 1860–1894" (Ph.D. thesis, University of Adelaide).

Maddock, K., 1972. *The Australian Aborigines: A Portrait of Their Society.* (London : Allen Lane/Penguin).

Meggitt, M. J., 1955. "Djanba Among the Walbiri, Central Australia", *Anthropos* 50 : 375–403.

——, 1962. *Desert People* (Sydney : Angus & Robertson).

Peterson, N., 1970. "Bulawandi: A Central Australian Ceremony for the Resolution of Conflict", in *Australian Aboriginal Anthropology*, ed. R. M. Berndt (Nedlands : University of Western Australia Press), pp. 200–15.

Reid, J. C., 1978. "The Role of the *Marrnggitj* in Contemporary Health Care", *Oceania* 49, no. 2 : 96–109.

Spencer, W. B., and Gillen, F. J., 1899. *The Native Tribes of Central Australia* (New York : Dover; repr. 1968).

Strehlow, T. G. H., 1971. *Songs of Central Australia* (Sydney : Angus & Robertson).

10
The Mabarn *and the Hospital: The Selection of Treatment in a Remote Aboriginal Community*

Myrna Tonkinson

In this paper, the selection of treatment in the Western Desert Aboriginal community of Jigalong is discussed. Investigations were carried out during ten months in 1974, followed by a ten-week period in 1978–79.[1] During both field periods, a number of people were interviewed about illness, its causes, the methods of treatment and their efficacy, the work of traditional healers (*mabarn*) and of the doctors and nurses. In the second field season, detailed records were kept of episodes of illness and treatment in five households, representing forty-eight individuals, over an eight-week period, and of other episodes of individual illness. People were consulted about health-related matters, the hospital was visited several times each week, talks were held with patients and with the sisters in charge, and *mabarn* were observed at work whenever the opportunity arose.

Some five hundred Aborigines and twenty Europeans make up the Jigalong community. The population fluctuated greatly during the summer of 1978–79, as almost a third of the Aboriginal residents went away to Balgo, Strelley and Wiluna for ceremonies or to visit relatives; conversely, visitors from those settlements sometimes swelled the Jigalong population.

TREATMENT OPTIONS

The community is served by a small out-patient hospital, usually staffed by two European nursing sisters (though in the 1978–79 summer, a single sister was in charge most of the time), assisted by one Aboriginal man employed on a full-time basis and three Aboriginal women who work part-time. These four Aboriginal workers are trained on the job. There are two untrained Aboriginal "camp nurses", who dispense non-prescription drugs and give first-aid, especially at the weekends. Once a week, a doctor flies in to conduct a clinic. The hospital is used heavily by the community. The sisters are so busy with the treatment of illness and injury that there is little time for any preventive activity, other than immunization of children. During the 1978–79 fieldwork period, figures were obtained on the number of encounters per week for three weeks. The weekly average was ninety-four. On the days when a doctor was present, the number of patients seen was 60 per cent higher than on other days.

The community is served also by several *mabarn* (traditional doctors). These men have the power to explain and cure illness. They also can influence the weather, chase away evil spirits and restore order in other ways. There are fourteen practising *mabarn* residing at Jigalong. (One of the more active Jigalong *mabarn* was absent for most of the 1978–79 visit.)

Mabarn from other communities visited Jigalong during this time, and each treated some of the sick. Not all *mabarn* are called upon with equal frequency for treatment, nor do they all respond with equal willingness to requests for their services. However, seven Jigalong *mabarn* and three visitors were observed at work, some on a number of occasions. Numerous reports also were recorded on the activities and accomplishments of various *mabarn*.

While it is much more difficult to check on the number of medical treatments dispensed by *mabarn* than by hospital staff, it was apparent that there were several such sessions most days at Jigalong.

In addition to the two major healing services, members of the Jigalong community use a variety of non-specialist healing methods to treat themselves and each other. The most common of these are:

(a) *Red ochre (budjurr) and fat applications for pain and fever:* Ochre is considered to be a potent medicine because it is believed to be the metamorphosed blood of ancestral beings. It is combined with fat and applied to painful areas of the body and is thought to be effective internally as well as externally. The mixture may be applied over an area where there is internal pain. An ochre-fat mixture — or fat alone (goanna fat is thought to be especially good, but dripping from the community store is used more often) — is considered to have a cooling effect and is applied when there is fever. "Cooling" applies not only to lowering temperature, but more generally to neutralizing illness. Ochre is so potent that it is used sparingly on children. For infants, it is applied only lightly over the fontanel. The efficacy of the ochre-fat mixture is greatly enhanced if it is prepared and sung-over in the "bush" (men's or women's secret ritual grounds). It may be applied in the bush or brought back to camp and used there. In this form, it is not used on children. Ochre-fat mixture also is applied as a preventive medicine.

(b) *Massage:* Although *mabarn* often use massage as part of their treatment, it also is used by non-specialists. It may or may not be used in combination with ochre and fat.

(c) *Binding:* Hair string or cloth is used to bind the head for headache, often in combination with the application of ochre and fat.

(d) *Sponging:* Sponging with water or the placing of damp cloths on the head or body are sometimes employed to combat fever. These techniques are used especially with children.

(e) *Plant medicines:* These are used in the form of infusions, which are drunk or applied externally. This form of treatment is used only when other methods have been unsuccessful and when the patient's condition is considered to be serious. This may be due to the fact that medical plants are not found within the settlement and special effort must be made to obtain them. The pharmacopoeia is small and many of the old people aver that they did not use plant medicines in the desert, except for one type, which was chewed and used to treat wounds and sores. The plants that *are* used today are considered to be highly potent medicines. Two or three individuals at Jigalong are said to be particularly knowledgeable about plant medicines, but there are no specialists, and individuals may use medicinal plants in their own ways.

(f) *Urine:* Urine sometimes is used medicinally by some old people. It is caught in a container and placed in the sun, then drunk or poured in the nostrils or ears. This treatment is used for colds and congestion.

(g) *Analgesics:* Analgesics are available from the store and are purchased by some people.

THE CHOICE OF TREATMENT OPTIONS

The methods of treatment outlined above are used with varying frequency. There is no simple, easily predicted "hierarchy of resort" (Romanucci-Ross, 1969). However, it is possible to draw conclusions from ethnographic observations, as well as from statistical data about the selection of treatment.

People at Jigalong respond in a variety of ways to the onset of illness. Some suffer in silence; some discuss their discomfort but take no action; some rest and await recovery; some seek some other form of treatment.

Self-administered remedies are widely used, but this may not mean that the illness is considered trivial; nor are home remedies necessarily the first resort. Plant medicines generally are used for serious complaints, usually after the patient has sought treatment from both Aboriginal and European specialists.

Not everyone uses all types of treatment with equal frequency. For example, older people who fear being sent away to hospital may conceal their illness from the medical authorities and seek relief from home remedies or from a *mabarn*. On the other hand, many young people tend to use the hospital rather than home cures. However, even the most "acculturated" young people will express faith in the healing power of *mabarn*, and even the most "traditional" old people sometimes seek pain-killing drugs from the nurse or doctor. Criticism either of the hospital-based services or the *mabarn* is uncommon. When it does occur, the criticism is of personalities and attitudes, and sometimes of the perceived competence of the practitioners, but seldom of the overall efficacy of the method of treatment. A few skeptics may be reluctant to use some treatments, but even they consult doctors and *mabarn* if really ill. One man who spoke disparagingly of the ability of either practitioners to help him, met with vehement disagreement from his wives. On the several occasions his wives brought a *mabarn* to treat him, he did not resist. The same man also would ask others to get medication from the hospital for him.

The type of illness may influence the choice of treatment. For example, wounds, sores, minor aches and pains will be taken to the hospital for treatment. Exceptions include spear wounds, which sometimes are concealed from the medical authorities. Sudden symptoms, particularly in children, are referred to the *mabarn*, regardless of what other measures are taken. Symptoms such as diarrhoea or sharp pain may be treated by the hospital and/or *mabarn*. Chronic and acute conditions almost invariably are treated by a combination of methods — in succession, or more commonly, contemporaneously — the most frequent combination is use of the *mabarn* and the hospital, sometimes with the addition of home remedies.

The table below summarizes 56 illness episodes from the 5 households recorded over a period of 8 weeks. It reveals the tend-

	No Treatment	Home Remedies	*Mabarn*	Hospital	Combination	Total
No.	3	7	9	19[a]	18	56
%	5.4	12.5	16.1	33.9	32.1	100

(a) Of these, 9 (16% of the total) were wounds, boils, broken bones or sore eyes or ears. As noted above, such complaints usually are referred to the hospital.

ency for people to use a combination of treatment methods for a high proportion of illnesses.

Reasons other than assessments of the efficacy of the available treatments and expected results influence choice. Factors affecting the choice of specialists include the following:

(a) The ease of obtaining a particular treatment influences choice. For example, in one case recorded, a child with diarrhoea, who was restless and crying in the night, was treated by her father, although he is not a fully fledged *mabarn.* (He is said to have the power, but he is still young and does not normally treat anyone.) Another member of the household said that this was done because it was late at night and it was more convenient to take this action than go to the hospital or seek a practising *mabarn.* The child got some relief and slept through the night, and was taken to the hospital the next day.

(b) A *mabarn* works out in the open and members of the patient's family and others who are interested can watch him work. Usually he makes comments as he works about what he finds and expresses his thoughts as to the cause of the problem. Conversely, a doctor or nurse treats the patient in private and those who are not sick are discouraged from entering the clinic. Therefore, if the illness is one about which the patient wants reassurance from family and friends, as well as from the healer, he or she may consult a *mabarn.* If the illness is something a patient wishes to keep secret, he or she may choose hospital treatment.

(c) *Mabarn* prefer not to treat people in the heat of the day, and therefore people who are anxious to have immediate relief may go to the hospital. Conversely, the hospital is closed in the evening, at which time the *mabarn* are more likely to be available. This is not an invariable situation, since *mabarn* sometimes do work during the day and people sometimes do go to the sisters at night for treatment.

(d) The *mabarn* is well known to the patient, while the European doctor is a stranger, who comes and goes. Sisters, though resident in the community, seldom stay for more than a few months. Confidence in these practitioners varies accordingly.

In order to explain the process of selection of treatment in Jigalong, it is necessary to discuss the characteristics of traditional doctors and the beliefs people hold about the causes of illness and its remedies.

THE MABARN

A number of researchers have described traditional healers and their role and status in Aboriginal societies (e.g. Berndt, 1964; Cawte, 1974; Eastwell, 1973; Reid, 1978; and most notably, Elkin, 1977). Many of the general characteristics of "medicine-men" are true of Jigalong healers, but some differences are worthy of note here. (See also Tonkinson, 1978 : 106–9, for details on Western Desert *mabarn*.)

In the languages spoken at Jigalong, the word *mabarn* refers both to the people who have healing powers and the source of that power. The sources are magical objects, usually kept in the stomach, or less commonly in the arms, thigh or head of the *mabarn* and removed for use in curing or (if they have evil intentions) harming others (Tonkinson, 1974 : 78). The word *mabarn* can connote any unusual power and the possessor thereof, but most commonly refers to those persons who have the wisdom and skill to use extraordinary human and non-human powers to diagnose and treat illness and, sometimes, to influence the weather. *Mabarn* also help to maintain order and social control in the community through their curing activities.

Almost all of the fourteen *mabarn* at Jigalong are middle-aged men and old men. (A notable exception is a young man, the son of a practising *mabarn*, who has been treating people since he was a child.) Not all *mabarn* are equally active, because illness and age are said to weaken the powers of *mabarn* temporarily or permanently. Such *mabarn* are more responsive to requests and some are in greater demand than others. In addition to the active and generally acknowledged practitioners, there are at least five young men and boys who are recognized by their relatives and others as having the powers of *mabarn*, but who as yet are not practising because they are too young.

Qualifications

Most *mabarn* at Jigalong are sons or brothers' sons of other *mabarn*. It is generally agreed that most *mabarn* are born with their power; it is *djugurdanidjanu* ("from the dreamtime"). When asked, *mabarn* will say they were *mabarn* before they took on human form. Thus there is no direct patrilineal inheritance of these powers, but the powers are associated with certain sites and certain ancestral beings, and since a son shares his father's country and sometimes ancestral totems as well, it is not surprising that these powers occur among men related to each other as brothers or fathers and sons. The ancestral totem is the dreamtime being(s) from whose spiritual essence a person is derived. It is acquired by birth "in the vicinity of the route of the particular ancestral being or group of beings" (Tonkinson, 1974 : 76). Occasionally a man who was not born a *mabarn* acquires power directly from a *mabarn*, and one *mabarn* can acquire additional power from another (R. Tonkinson, pers. comm.).

Although there are reports of female Aboriginal healers elsewhere in Australia (Berndt, 1964; Reid, 1978) and although the women of Jigalong and Warrabri (Bell, in this volume) perform healing rituals, there are no female *mabarn* at Jigalong. Some people acknowledge that a woman can have these powers because they know of women in other places who do, but it is considered unusual for women to be *mabarn*. One old *mabarn* stated emphatically that women cannot be *mabarn*, and suggested that this is because they are without a penis. Another *mabarn* said there used to be female *mabarn*, but shortly after the group settled at Jigalong, there was an epidemic in which many people died and the women lost the power to be *mabarn*. There is no consistent explanation for the absence of female *mabarn*.

A boy thought to have been born with *mabarn* power can display certain characteristics in childhood that indicate this. His father or some other *mabarn* will notice something about his hands or his manner that denotes his talent (cf. Elkin, 1977 : 15). However, the posession of this power is thought to be potentially dangerous to children, and therefore its use usually is delayed until the boy reaches adulthood. Sometimes a child's power is cut off altogether by his father because it is thought to be too great and therefore too dangerous (cf. Reid, 1978). It is more common for a young man with *mabarn* power to pass through some of the stages of initiation and to be a married adult before his power is released by another *mabarn* — "his hands are opened". However, before this actually occurs, a young *mabarn* may start to practise because he "feels" an urge to do so. This tends to happen when someone is ill and no established *mabarn* is available.

Techniques

Touching is fundamental to the work of a *mabarn*. The verb "to touch" (*bambula*) is used when describing what a *mabarn* does.

People say of an effective healer that "he has a good hand". *Mabarn* are said to keep various objects inside their bodies and pull them out as they work. They insert curing objects into the bodies of their patients, remove sorcery objects from the bodies of victims, all with the vigorous use of their hands. In addition, the *mabarn* use massage to heal and relieve pain and discomfort. Pressure is applied to the head and other parts of the body to dispel pain.

Sucking is another significant *mabarn* technique. Many *mabarn* will suck a part of a patient's body, usually the chest or abdominal area. The sucking seems to draw blood and this then is spat into a container. This blood is examined for sorcery objects thought to have been "fired" at the victim from a distance, to cause sickness. Sometimes water is added to the blood and it is left in the open for a while, then discarded. This action is said to cool the patient down. The notions that heat is associated with illness and that sick people need internal cooling are pervasive, but Aborigines at Jigalong do not elaborate.

Each *mabarn* has one or more spirit familiars who assist him in healing. These familiars reside at particular sites in the traditional country of the healer, but can be summoned when needed. One man at Jigalong has a small bird as his main familiar. This bird usually is available to help him and especially to assist him in diagnosing illness. However, it retreats to its country whenever he is weakened by illness or worry, and returns again when he is well and strong.

Dreaming is another technique available to *mabarn* as an aid to diagnosis and curing. The healer may travel in a dream to the site from which his power originates; he may take with him an organ of the patient's body that requires cleansing. Sometimes he makes contact with his familiar(s) in dreams and thus consults them as to the cause and/or cure for an illness. One of the *mabarn* at Jigalong works only through dreams — he does not "touch" patients, rather he "dreams" for them. Another *mabarn* has a lame arm and though not able to do much touching, still is considered powerful. This man also uses dreams. In one case, he was asked by a sick woman for help. He slept outside her house for one night and had a dream that showed him the cause of her illness. Those *mabarn* who regularly use touch also rely on dreams as an important part of their work. One man who has power but does not practise, said that when he is ill, he usually treats himself rather than consulting another *mabarn*. This he accomplishes by returning magically to his country. In sleep, he turns himself into a woman and travels through the air with the aid of an object shaped like a boomerang. In his own country, he encounters a mythological snake-woman who is associated with a site for which he is responsible. The snake-woman takes him into the ground and up again, and he is restored to health. Sometimes he takes one of his brothers with him by placing the brother (in his dream) in his stomach.

Apart from the small objects of stone, shell or wood that they are said to keep within their bodies and which are sources of their power, the *mabarn* have no curing paraphernalia.

TREATMENT CONDITIONS

Mabarn work alone, except when the patient is thought to be gravely ill. In such cases, several *mabarn* may treat the sick person simultaneously. Sometimes up to six *mabarn* may work together on a patient. They discuss the situation among themselves, but each adopts his own style of treatment. For example, one *mabarn* may concentrate on imparting strength to the patient by removing power from his own body and pressing it into the patient; another may go back and forth between the patient and a place in the open, from which he faces the direction of his country and consults with his spirit helper(s). *Mabarn* almost always talk to the patient (even when the patient is unconscious) during treatment. They also talk to the relatives and others who are present. They may enlist the assistance of these onlookers to hold or move the patient.

The work of the *mabarn* requires energy and concentration, and they use their curing skills judiciously. They talk of their power as something that waxes and wanes, and which can be used effectively only under ideal conditions. Most important of these is that the *mabarn* himself should be in good physical health to be able to restore others to health. Thus a *mabarn* who is feeling ill will avoid treating others. He may say that he is feeling "weak" or that his power is "light", and therefore he is unable to respond to a request for help. There are two old *mabarn* at Jigalong who appear to be in good health, but who claim frequently that they have lost their power to heal. Nevertheless, the sick often call upon them for treatment. These old men may refuse, but they usually can be prevailed upon to attempt a cure. It is thought that any *mabarn* may become temporarily unable to cure effectively, but it is rare for a *mabarn* to lose his power altogether. The power of the *mabarn* is enduring. "That old bloke may be deaf now, but he is still good; he is a strong *mabarn*." "His arm is no good any more; he can't do much, but he is a *mabarn* just the same; he has helped me lots of times."

Mood is also a factor that influences the action of the *mabarn*. He may refuse to treat a patient because he does not feel like it, or because he is preoccupied with some other task. Such a refusal may evoke anger in the person seeking healing, and therefore it may be that the *mabarn* proffers the more acceptable excuse that he is feeling weak or light.

Certain environmental conditions also are considered desirable for the work of *mabarn*. As noted earlier, *mabarn* avoid treating people during the day. They imply that treatment will not be very effective if administered when the weather is very hot. This may be related to the view that illness is associated with heat inside the body. Healing is done outdoors. The only time that *mabarn* work indoors is when the patient is in hospital and is too ill to be moved.

The *mabarn* will work in a variety of settings. Sometimes the patient goes to him and is treated in his camp. Often he will go to the patient's camp. It is becoming increasingly common to find a *mabarn* working around the hospital — and, on occasion, in it — with the knowledge and sometimes approval of the medical staff. *Mabarn* also refer patients to the hospital for further treatment, especially when symptoms are severe or persistent.

DIAGNOSIS AND TREATMENT

After examining and talking with the patient, and perhaps consulting his spirit familiar on the spot or in a dream, the healer offers an explanation for the illness. The presence of foreign objects in the body is offered as the most common cause of illness. Such objects take a variety of forms. Pieces of shell, wire or stones often are "extracted" from the patient's body and shown to the patient and onlookers as proof that the sufferer has been a victim of sorcery. These objects are said to have been sent flying into the victim's body, usually from some distant place. Other foreign objects are seen by the *mabarn* in dreams and are not shown. One man who said he was "very sick" and was hearing noises, was told by the *mabarn* that he saw in a dream a miniature version of a flagon about to enter the man and make him sick. The *mabarn* captured the flagon and wedged it in a fork in a tree. The patient recovered the next day, and gave up drinking.

In another case, a *mabarn* reported that he had "seen" in a dream a bearded, clothed miniature man inside the stomach of a sick woman, whose stomach was greatly distended. He said that another *mabarn* had fired a sorcery object into the woman's body and made the object turn into himself. Still in the dream, the Jigalong *mabarn* twirled a lighted stick against the soles of the woman's feet and the heat went to the woman's stomach and caused the sorcerer to flee.

After this, the woman felt "lighter" (R. Tonkinson, pers. comm.).

Another common diagnosis is that a body organ has sores on it, holes in it or has been burned. In such cases, the *mabarn* may "remove" the organ while the patient is asleep and take it away to the site where his power rests, for cleansing and curing.

People sometimes are told that they will recover quickly. Sometimes they are told they are very ill and it will be a long time before they are better. Seldom are they told they will not recover at all. The *mabarn* may refer serious cases to other *mabarn* he considers more powerful or more able to help.

If the sickness persists, a patient may make repeated visits to one or more *mabarn* for massage, sucking or removal of objects. But *mabarn* give few directives for continuing treatment. Sometimes certain foods are recommended or proscribed: for example, a patient may be told to eat plains-kangaroo meat to built up his strength or to avoid emu meat.

CLIENTELE

A *mabarn* usually treats his own relatives, consanguineal and affinal, and certain countrymen. People seeking treatment usually approach a *mabarn* in a nearby camp first, since residence is based on kinship and affinity. The doctor is therefore most likely to be a relative well known to the patient. However, there is no prohibition on consulting a distant *mabarn*, and this often occurs when there is serious illness. Almost any member of the community is able to choose from among a few *mabarn* from within his extended family and countrymen, and some people have very definite preferences. Two or three healers have a reputation for producing successful results and thus have more clients than others. Usually young children are treated by "grandfathers", who are said to be especially concerned about the health of their small relatives. A *mabarn* does not treat people with whom he has an avoidance relationship (cf. Reid, 1978 : 105), although this rule may be dispensed with when the illness is critical. It is thought by some that the most effective treatment a very sick woman can receive is from a "son-in-law", despite the strict avoidance relationship. In one case observed, a woman covered her face with a rag while a son-in-law treated her. In another case where the patient was dying and was unconscious, no effort was made by others to shield her face from her "son-in-law's" view.

PAYMENT

The services of *mabarn* are highly valued, but are not rewarded necessarily by payment. A *mabarn* treats his sick relatives and countrymen as part of his kin obligations. Similarly, those whom he treats may offer gifts of money or goods as their part of the chain of reciprocity. When asked whether they compensate *mabarn* for treatment, it is common for people to respond along the lines of: "No, I don't pay him, he's my uncle" or "He doesn't want money, he's her grandfather." But people sometimes state the principle of reciprocity, which affects their relationship with *mabarn*. Thus one woman explained: "I give [him] money, sometimes $5, $10, and I give him food because he is my 'father' and I know he will touch me and my children. But I don't *pay* him really."

There is no strict schedule of payments for the services of *mabarn* and there is wide variation in the amount and type of payment. Money is the most common form of compensation and people mention fees of from $2 to $20. When someone is very ill and both patient and relatives want a *mabarn* to make a special effort on their behalf, they may make a large payment to the *mabarn*. In such cases, there are reports of families pooling funds to pay for treatment by one or several *mabarn*. The fee for service is paid when the patient goes outside his kin group for treatment or, occasionally, when the *mabarn* is a relative who demands payment. People also bestow gifts on *mabarn* out of gratitude for successful treatment, or as an ongoing insurance against the possible need for treatment in the future.

THE CAUSES OF ILLNESS

People at Jigalong acknowledge several causes of illness. However, symptoms cannot be readily categorized.

Environmental factors such as excessive heat or cold may cause colds, aches and other maladies. In the summer of 1978–79, many children suffered diarrhoea, vomiting, coughs and colds; women remarked that this was because it was very hot. To many older Jigalong residents, the settlement itself is an unhealthy place compared with the desert. Prolonged illness with such symptoms invariably would lead to people searching for other explanations, however.

Powerful emotions also are seen to cause illness. Loss of appetite, weight loss, listlessness and pain are symptoms that are sometimes attributed to emotional causes. *Yundiri* (resentment, sulking) is by far the emotion most frequently linked to illness; in fact, a synonym for *yundiri* is *wirla walygurini* (the stomach becoming bad/sick). Some women expressed the view that men are more prone than women to become ill from *yundiri*. *Gunda* (shame, embarrassment) also may lead to sickness. With lesser frequency, worry, homesickness, grief and jealousy are said to be causes of illness.

Magical causes of illness are a fundamental part of the aetiology to which Jigalong people subscribe and are crucial to an understanding of the selection of treatment. While humans and other beings can cause illness and death, and any acute or chronic illness that does not respond to treatment will be suspected of being magically induced, illness seldom will be initially attributed to these causes. Although sorcery or other "unnatural" causes may be suspected, they are only confirmed after the patient has failed to respond to a variety of treatments.

Magical causes of illness (and death) fall into several categories. Most serious illness and deaths are explained as due to sorcery. *Mabarn* are thought to have the power to kill as well as cure, but it is unusual to hear people voice suspicion of the local *mabarn* as practitioners of sorcery. Sorcerers are said to attack people either for personal reasons or under contract to enemies of the victim. For example, there are many stories of "big *mabarn*" who frequent the Port Hedland hospital in search of victims. (Jigalong people are suspicious of coastal people and others with whom they have no substantial links). Victims are killed, then revived, and then later die in hospital or after returning home. Some *mabarn* with evil proclivities are said to cause women to fall ill if they refuse their sexual advances. Angered relatives of a dead person, a wronged spouse and/or his or her relatives and others with grudges may engage one or more *mabarn* to take revenge on their behalf by causing the wrong-doer to fall ill or die. When someone is ill, it is quite common for that person and his family to consider whether they have incurred the wrath of someone who may have retaliated by using sorcery. Sorcerers are said to attack their victims by hurling a sorcery object through the air from a distance. Such attacks can go awry and hit the wrong person; they also can happen to small children, who are not otherwise potential victims of sorcery.

There is a particular type of sorcerer called *djinagarbil* (featherfeet), the thought of whom invokes great fear in people of all ages at Jigalong. These men travel great distances and enter the community usually under cover of darkness, find their victim, who must be alone and some distance from the camp, stun him, then remove one or more organs or insert a lethal object into his body. They then revive the victim, who returns to the camp and quickly sickens and dies. *Djinagarbil* attack people for a variety of reasons:

they may be taking revenge, imposing punishment for ritual infractions, or making random attacks on the unwary. When an old woman died of heat exhaustion away from the settlement, one pervasive explanation was that she had run into *djinagarbil* as she walked alone, looking for her husband, who had gone to find water. The husband, a *mabarn*, said he had seen *djinagarbil* in the area.

Spirit beings can cause illness and death deliberately or accidentally. *Gurdi* (spirits of the dead) are said to like to hover around a camp, to be close to their relatives. Such spirits are not malevolent, they merely seek company. However, they can be dangerous to the relatives and others, and this is why a camp is vacated after a death. Children and close relatives are especially susceptible, particularly at night or early morning.

Marlbu are malevolent spirits that attack people who wander into their territory. *Marlbu* inhabit some sacred and dangerous sites, and it is not safe for anyone to enter these places in person or during dream spirit travels, unless accompanied by a *mabarn* who is familiar with the area. *Marlbu* also visit a settlement at night and will harm those they encounter. Such attacks can lead to illness or death.

The loss of the *nunu* (soul) is another cause of illness, and is one to which children are especially susceptible. The symptoms that indicate this loss are the head falling limply, the eyes rolling or the eyelids drooping. A *mabarn* is needed to restore the soul. One woman told of being in hospital with her two-year-old son and noticing these symptoms. She immediately took him from the hospital (without notifying anyone there) to a nearby settlement, where a *mabarn* restored his soul, thus saving him from death.

Jigalong people believe that victims of sorcery have suffered attacks on their internal organs, particularly the liver and kidneys. When a European diagnosis such as cancer is given by hospital staff, it is seen as a confirmation of the assumed condition of "something bad inside". People sometimes quote the doctor's description of such a condition as part of the evidence for sorcery.

Symptoms such as difficulty with elimination and loss of appetite are viewed with alarm because they indicate something wrong internally. The relatives of a woman who was unconscious and said by the Flying Doctor to be dying, asked anxiously whether she had been fed while she was in hospital in Perth. They were disturbed by the fact that the sisters were not making any attempt to feed her.

Essential to curing then are getting rid of the "bad stuff" from inside and restoring the normal functioning of the body. *Mabarn* may suck out this "bad stuff" and patients may take emetics so that they can vomit up the "bad stuff".

CONCLUSIONS

Given the Jigalong people's beliefs about the causes of illness and in the special powers of the *mabarn*, it is not surprising that in any cases of prolonged or serious illness, the *mabarn* will play an important part in the curing. Because *mabarn* can offer an explanation for a condition based on a theory of illness that is understood by the patient and those concerned for the welfare of the patient, he is able to provide comfort and reassurance. A European doctor may offer an explanation of an illness, but this is seldom meaningful to Aboriginal patients, who continue to feel the need for further specialist help. Supportive communication is part of the style of the *mabarn*. He almost never declares a case hopeless and constantly assures patients that they are getting better.

Combating the effects of sorcery is a continuing, vital part of the work of *mabarn*. As one woman put it: "If you get sick from *mardu* (human) [i.e. if you are a sorcery victim], no [European] doctor can help you, only *mabarn* can make you better." The *mabarn* may or may not succeed in curing a sorcery victim. It depends on how powerful he is compared to the sorcerer, and how quickly the victim seeks his help. No amount of treatment by medical personnel can substitute for the treatment delivered by a *mabarn*, who alone can discover the real cause of the illness.

Premature death or chronic illness usually are blamed either on the evil actions of others or on neglect of symptoms by patients and their close relatives, rather than on poor care from *mabarn* or medical people. By relating illness to the behaviour of the patient and/or close relatives of the patient, the *mabarn* plays a subtle role in social control. Since the community accepts that "bad" behaviour — such as abandoning a spouse, marrying wrongly, breaking ritual taboos or heavy drinking — can lead to the illness of parents or other relatives, the *mabarn* need only reinforce this view when explaining *why* a patient is ill.

Remarkable recoveries are invariably attributed to the power of *mabarn*, even when the patient has received medical treatment as well. While different *mabarn* may give varied diagnoses of an illness and *mabarn* diagnoses may differ from that of the medical staff, such discrepancies are not seen as contradictory but as part of one larger explanation, or primacy is given to the diagnosis of a "big" or "strong" *mabarn*.

Notwithstanding the fact that peoply rely heavily on their own medical resources at Jigalong, traditional Aboriginal medicine and European medicine coexist well. Both systems are used heavily by the Aboriginal residents, who perceive both as expert in providing cures, or at least relieving symptoms, for many ailments. The Aborigines do not see the two systems as conflicting, instead they use both according to their needs at a particular time. Sometimes one method of treatment is considered preferable (for example, the hospital for wounds, *mabarn* for "soul loss"). In situations where either method will suffice, people select the more convenient. There is no perceived contradiction in relying on both systems of curing at the same time.

When an illness is chronic or acute, people use all available treatments, sometimes going straight from a European specialist to an Aboriginal one, or vice versa. This tendency is strengthened by the fact that *mabarn* often refer patients to the hospital and, in recent years, some European medical staff refer patients to *mabarn* or consult with *mabarn* about difficult cases. I believe this trend is commendable, but there are limits to combining the two systems. While there are some advantages to the efforts in parts of Australia to train traditional doctors as health workers, or otherwise involve them in health services, this may undermine the role of Aboriginal healers, since it places them in an unfamiliar situation, where others are in charge. This trend also could result in limiting people's choices by making the role of the *mabarn* ambiguous.

In a community where morbidity and mortality are so high, the attitude of the Jigalong Aborigines is rational and understandable. They attempt to maximize their options for treatment for any illness. The availability of options does not, however, solve the health problems of this community. There is still a great need for improved living conditions and health services. Perhaps the greatest need of all is for improved communication between the European-Australian medical people and the Aborigines who are their patients: the lack of understanding of basic ideas and values, especially on the part of doctors and nurses, who do not question the imposition of their Western views of health and healing on Aborigines, can only exacerbate the already serious health problems of communities such as Jigalong.

NOTES

[1] The research on which this paper is based was made possible by grants (in 1974 and 1978) from the Australian Institute of Aboriginal Studies. Dr Robert Tonkinson made available to me his field notes on *mabarn*, collected during a number of field trips since 1963. He also conducted for me an interview with one Jigalong *mabarn* in January 1979. For valuable comments on an earlier draft of this paper, I am grateful to Dr Peter Ucko, Dr Janice Reid and Dr Alan Thorne. I am indebted to many people at Jigalong who provided the material on which this paper

is based. In particular, I thank Margaret Sailor, who spent many hours instructing me on these and other topics.

REFERENCES

Berndt, C. H., 1964. "The Role of Native Doctors in Aboriginal Australia", in *Magic, Faith and Healing*, ed. A. Kiev (New York : Free Press of Glencoe), pp. 264–82.

Cawte, J. E., 1974. *Medicine is the Law* (Honolulu : University Press of Hawaii).

Eastwell, H. D., 1973. "The Traditional Healer in Modern Arnhem Land", *Medical Journal of Australia* 2, no. 22 : 1011–17.

Elkin, A. P., 1977. *Aboriginal Men of High Degree* (St Lucia : Queensland University Press, 2nd edn); first published 1945.

Reid, J. C., 1978. "The Role of the *Marrnggitj* in Contemporary Health Care", *Oceania* 49, no. 2 : 96–109.

Romanucci-Ross, Lola, 1969. "The Hierarchy of Resort in Curative Practices: The Admiralty Islands, Melanesia", *Journal of Health and Social Behaviour* 10 : 201–9.

Tonkinson, R., 1970. "Aboriginal Dream Spirit Beliefs in a Contact Situation: Jigalong, Western Australia", in *Australian Aboriginal Anthropology*, ed. R. M. Berndt (Nedlands : University of W.A. Press), pp. 277–91.

——, 1974. *The Jigalong Mob: Aboriginal Victors of the Desert Crusade* (Menlo Park, Calif. : Cummings).

——, 1978. *The Mardudjara Aborigines: Living the Dream in Australia's Desert* (New York : Holt, Rinehart & Winston).